D1475159

SECOND EDITION

Say "Yes" To Love

God Unveils SoulMate Love and Sacred Sexuality

Through Yael and Doug Powell

SAY 'YES' TO LOVE,
God Unveils SoulMate Love and Sacred Sexuality
Through Yael and Doug Powell

Copyright 2002 by Yael and Doug Powell
Second Edition 2005

Paperback Original ISBN 0-9725991-1-8
Circle of Light Press

All rights reserved. All of any part of this publication may be reproduced by any means, electronic or mechanical, except for commercial purposes. Anyone other than book stores and book distributors who wishes to use this book in whole or in part for commercial purposes, may not do so without written permission from:

Yael and Doug Powell
CIRCLE OF LIGHT
3969 Mundell Road
Eureka Springs, AR 72631

Cover design and book layout by Judith Bicking
Compilation, editing of Messages by Shanna Mac Lean
Art work by Yael Powell

Web sites: www.circleoflight.net
www.unitingtwinflames.com
Email: connect@circleoflight.net

Printing: InstantPublisher.com Collierville, TN

SAY "YES" TO LOVE SERIES
through Yael and Doug Powell

Say "Yes" To Love, God Explains SoulMates
SECOND EDITION

Say "Yes" To Love, God Unveils SoulMate Love
and Sacred Sexuality
SECOND EDITION

Say "Yes" to Love, God's Guidance to LightWorkers

Say "Yes" to Love, God Leads Humanity
Toward Christ Consciousness

Say "Yes" to Love,
Magic Cat (an enlightened animal)
Explains Creation

In Process:

Say "Yes" to Love, Giving Birth to the Christ Light

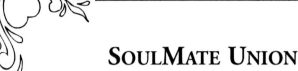

SOULMATE UNION

Foreword by Claire Heartsong

I am deeply honored to bring forth words that might inspire you to open your hearts to *Say "Yes" to Love: God Unveils Soulmate Love and Sacred Sexuality*. Never in the years since the pivotal turning point of Harmonic Convergence in 1987 have I found such powerful energies of SoulMate Love evoked and so clearly revealed. Within these pages and words are the very energies Divine Creator is using to bring every particle of Creation back Home. When these incomprehensible energies are allowed to permeate the heart of your every atom, Father-Mother-God promises that you will experience a shift in your perception. It is then that you will behold God as your very Self, your Beloved in eternal embrace. I assure you that the journey you are about to embark upon while reading these Messages will be that of a gentle return to your true self—a being of Love. Thus it is that your SoulMate will come forth —your mirror revealing you as the One Love. Together you shall remember the cosmic bridal chamber where your forever Union is creating all life.

Through Yael and Doug, our beloved Creator uses simple, yet empowering words of love, compassion and mirth that sparkle with the same brilliance that lights the night sky. The mysteries of SoulMate Love are illumined. Together, we turn away from the dark to face the light. Shadowy dramas of being separate no longer entertain. With singular purpose you, who choose to live and be the Love of God – the Christ – are inspired to remember how to give love freely as does the day's shining orb bless all upon its path. Bathed in orgasmic bliss, Father-Mother-God lavishes you and all Creation with the passionate ardor of a lover who never tires of Lovemaking. Remembering Sacred Sexuality as God's path to becoming Love again you may suddenly recognize your SoulMate as the one who shares your life and bed.

With a sense of urgency within each Now, God issues an ecstatic Call. This is the time we agreed to meet as SoulMates melded in a Union foreordained. As SoulMate couples, we are the torch of freedom that melts frozen hearts afraid to love. We are the promised Christ ascending Mother Earth. Blessed indeed are those who say "Yes" to Love!

Claire Heartsong is the author of *Anna, Grandmother of Jesus: A Message of Wisdom and Love* and the co-author of *St. Germain: Twin-Souls & Soulmates.* You can learn more about Claire by visiting her website:

www.shastaspirit.com/heartsong
http://www.shastaspirit.com/heartsong>
She can be contacted at annarose@xmission.com or claireheartsong@yahoo.com.

WORDS FROM READERS OF THE SAY "YES" TO LOVE SERIES

"I proceed very slowly reading these Messages because it's as if it weren't my eyes that were reading it, but my heart. It's as if I've just come Home. Your Messages are so 'soft.' I don't know how else to describe them. It feels like being wrapped in something very delicate. I keep crying all the time when I read them... I feel so very beloved." Paula Launonen, Ravenna, Italy

"Everything in the Messages resonates so deeply in me. I am amazed that I've found so much that had already been revealed to me in visions and dreams...it sometimes takes my breath away! It has given so much validity to everything I had already come to believe. Thank you all for feeling the need to share the Messages. They have meant so much to me in my journey. It's kind of like piloting a boat by the stars and one day discovering a secret compartment full of maps that show where all the ports of call are located. It makes it so much easier to get where you want to go!" Diane Dunville, Lanexa, VA

"Words are so inadequate to describe how these books have touched my life, especially God Explains SoulMates. It's what I always thought relationships can be, and I never found it put into black and white. Here it was, so perfectly described. I devoured it like I would the finest 'crème brule' not stopping until I had every last morsel of it, and then craved for more. It came at a time when I had said to my friends, 'I found my Twin Flame,' never knowing what it meant. Now I know." Carol Davis, Cat Spring, Texas

"In all my study, discernment, and spiritual practice over the years, I found that each teaching was only a step, only part of the process. I have known that each of us is so much more than our limited experiences have shown us. I seemed to need the bigger picture. I began to believe that I just was not ready or open enough to receive this divine manifestation. Then came Say 'YES' to Love. That grace, that grandness, that confirmation that we are so much more than we can ever imagine sang out to me boldly. The whole of co-creation was simplified and resonated fully within me. The consistent theme is that we are truly only Love and are much more than we can now comprehend. Say 'YES' to Love is also very practical — most notably in how to function in a world of duality when you know only Love is real. Just as the pressure of others' duality began eroding my knowing, this book arrived to help gently guide me. Just as Creator promised." Peggy Zetler, Dillon, Montana.

"These Messages are stunning, clear, beautiful, re-activating, stirring to the core of my being. This material reminds me of Home, reminds me to express the totality of my being, reminds me of how close to Home we are now, reminds me of my Twin Flame. Just having the books and knowing their content is a small sign of the ecstasy to come." Karen Porrit, U.K.

"These Messages, faithfully documented by Yael Powell, were brought to me at just the right time in my life and served as validation of what my Twin Flame and I had discovered on our own, without any outside influence. I can speak personally on the validity of this Twin Flame relationship as I was blessed enough in my lifetime to have been with my Twin Flame. Our story is for another time and another place, but it is important to state without qualification that the reality of the soulmate bond as expressed through God's Messages is not a fabrication or an idealistic view of what love can be... It is the greatest love that can be, the love of our Creator to us, and the ability to experience that kind of love within our soulmate bond." Rev. Adelle Tilton, The Church of Interfaith Christians, NE

DEDICATION

We dedicate this book to God, Who with tender Love has guided us in the unfoldment of our SoulMate Love, Who has gifted us with magnificent communion that in the mirror of each other's eyes, we truly know God's Love. In awe and Love and reverence, we pray to do, to live and to be only the Will of God.

We dedicate this book to all the precious hearts of humanity, with our prayer that their SoulMate's Love will create for each a heaven on Earth and usher in the New World.

We dedicate this book to Shanna, whose beautiful heart, amazing mind and nimble fingers have made this work a physical reality. Her Love, support and recognition have changed our lives, moving this work from knowing to accomplishing. Her presence in our life is a daily message from God affirming who we are together and catalyzing these messages into print.

And we dedicate this book to Pra, Shanna's Twin Flame (SoulMate), whose assistance from beyond this dimension has raised our vision continually, and whose Love has helped us anchor the patterning for Sacred Sexuality on Earth. His presence is an affirmation forever of the greater vision God has for our lives — far beyond all our seeming hurts and tragedies.

In Memoriam

In loving memory of Susan Lee Solar,
best friend, wild woman, explorer, adventurer and pioneer,
who was always looking for the highest vision of Love.
She is with her SoulMate now.

TABLE OF CONTENTS

PART ONE: SOULMATE LOVE

PART TWO: SACRED SEXUALITY

ACKNOWLEDGEMENTS

I first acknowledge my beloved Doug, my SoulMate, whom I love more deeply every day. Doug's increasing light and clarity is a continual inspiration to me and to all who know him. We have truly walked every step of this path together, from being two individuals full of fear and ego, to recognizing our SoulMate relationship and claiming daily more of the passion, beauty and ecstasy that God keeps lovingly showing us. I am so deeply grateful to God for tenderly unveiling to me my magnificent SoulMate, Doug.

Next to Doug, Shanna is my truest Soul Family. Shanna is mentioned in the Dedication, yet I have to say more. Shanna has not only catalyzed these books into print. She has held up a divine mirror of pure Love and shown me my true self. Thanks to her I have finally completely accepted the gift of bringing forth these Messages. I have moved beyond the fear of ego that kept me hidden, afraid to come forth, lest I "think too much of myself." Through Shanna's Love, I came to see myself with enough clarity that God could show me how the "trickster" ego can use even "humility" to keep us from totally giving our lives in service! Shanna is the most pure, light-filled being I have ever met. That God brought her "miraculously" into our lives in order to bring forth these Messages is one of our greatest gifts. Until Shanna I have never before known anyone whose life, dedication and Love of God so closely reflected my own. Though God is the author of these Messages, it is Shanna's hands that have shaped them into books.

I acknowledge my beautiful Soul Sister, Michelle, whose glorious voice and loving heart are also dedicated to bringing forth the vision of what this world is meant to be. The music of the spheres is her inspiration. The star-studded sky is her cathedral. She embodies all that is pure and perfect on the Earth. I am honored to share this path of service with her, and forever to be her friend.

I thank our sweet Mary, whose life belongs totally to God, for typing these Messages and blessing them with her Love. May she ever be a part of the Team, being grown and nourished as we are by these Messages.

Geoff and Leslie Oelsner and Jim and Lorraine May are my dearest and longest friends. Their support and Love mean everything to me. Cynthia and Tom Morin, although newer in my life, are definitely part of my spiritual family. With their enthusiasm for life, their dedication to the light and truth and their joyful loving hearts, they are a great blessing in my life.

I deeply thank Suzanne Muller, the woman who saved my life by taking me from the absolute terror of a life filled with sexual and physical abuse and horrible darkness. Suzanne placed my feet upon the Path of Light by teaching me to meditate thirty years ago, thus establishing in my life the spiritual practice which has ultimately brought forth these Messages.

I acknowledge Bernadine Greer, the most generous and most beautiful light I have ever known. Bernadine was in my life in the early years of coping with such disability that I could barely move. She would sit with me by my bed for hours, bathing me in Love and most especially giving me hope. Bernadine is no longer on the physical plane. I think of her often and sometimes feel her presence. It is with glad heart that I picture her watching over me.

To everyone who has touched my life, I give thanks!

Yael

Although sometimes it seems we are doing this all alone, at other times there is help there at every turn. There have been some amazing role models in my life. First and foremost are my parents, Art and Betty Powell. After 60 years of marriage, they are still in Love and so very supportive of each other. True SoulMates!

My three brothers and sister are all also in loving relationships. Some of them have raised families and some of them are now grandparents. All of them are dedicated partners.

I also acknowledge the Eureka Springs Mens' Council. For twelve years and counting, they have been there for me and for each other, through everything.

My mentor, Coach Molly Seeligson, has probably been the most significant influence during my transition phase. She assisted me as I moved from an entrepreneur, a businessman, a workaholic to a truly dedicated SoulMate and husband. It was difficult for me to let go of who I thought I was so that I could become who I was meant to be.

To everyone else, I thank you and bless you for the role you have played in assisting me to grow into who I have become.

Doug

INTRODUCTION

As I re-read these Messages in preparation for this book, I was filled with wonder and amazement. Though the Messages had come through me, I found myself learning new things and remembering things I had forgotten. I wrote notes to Shanna, our editor, on page after page saying, "This is fabulous!" Many times I found myself moved to tears. The tears were tears of joy at the beauty of these Messages and the power they have to transform all of us, and also tears of deep, profound gratitude for the incredible honor of being the vehicle through which God has given this gift.

If you will read with your heart, these Messages will do the same for you. They will fill you with awe and gratitude. And in ways both subtle and huge, on many levels in many ways, they will change you.

Please do not allow something like not having your SoulMate stop you from opening this book! In these pages God will reveal to you the amazing truth of Love and how it is already in your life. Step-by-step you will find the truth of your SoulMate and all the layers of resistance will melt away. There are blessings here for everyone, no matter what your current belief. Even if you don't immediately resonate with the Messages in this book, take it home and give it a place on your bookshelf. God has said that the radiation of this Love will open every heart in its proximity, and that even sitting on a bookshelf, it will do its work.

The honor of receiving this material under God's perfect tutelage really began when I met Doug, My SoulMate. I had begun to receive Messages from God two years earlier, and even before that time, I had experienced an amazing communion with nature, seeing the light that fed my garden and hearing what every plant wanted and needed.

At the time I began to receive the Messages from God, I had lost my physical mobility from a powerful disease. I was in great physical and emotional pain. I was very seriously considering ending my life. Through this dark night God reached forth with an incredible love and gave me the strength to continue. There was no doubt who was lifting me and renewing my faith in life. The Messages then were "flashes" of Love and of light. I would be wrapped in God's Divine Presence and given an "instant understanding" of some part of me that needed illumination. It was like receiving a "package" that was a totality. All the Love and information "dropped" all at once into my head. The understandings were like beacons and the Love sustained me as I gathered the fortitude to re-connect to life.

Then, on a December day in 1986 I sat for the first time with Doug, my new husband and the Love of my life. Although we had many a rocky road to travel ahead of us, even then we knew we were each other's destiny. I closed my eyes and touched Doug's hand. My entire being exploded into light – a loving, pulsing light that was alive with movement and luminosity. Dancing golden white particles shone all around me, merging together into a greater and greater light. The sense of Loving Presence grew, filled my heart and poured through me. My heart caught on fire. There is no other way to describe it. The fire leaped the gap between Doug and me and drew us together into an experience of becoming living flames ourselves, dancing together, "burning" in love and reaching higher and higher.

In the midst of this experience I reached for a notebook and pen and I wrote. As I wrote I was aware of being assisted with the energy, but I was also aware that, though illuminated by God's Love, I was doing my best with my words to describe that which is indescribable.

Thus these Messages began. They have now lovingly, unfailingly guided us through eighteen years of marriage. They have kept us going when we were ready to give up. They have explained ourselves to us. They have revealed to us our destiny. And as we have grown together as a result of God's tender guiding love, we have also grown in our ability to raise ourselves up to meet God at a higher level. In doing so, we have been greatly blessed with the understanding of the "piece" of information that it is our destiny to share.

In July of 2001 God brought us the joy of uniting with a key member of our Soul Family, Shanna. We had prayed that our next step for the Messages be revealed, along with the resources and people to bring it forth. Even before Shanna joined us at Circle of Light, we began a joint effort from a distance, our first book, *Say 'Yes' to Love, God Explains SoulMates*. When Shanna took up permanent residence at Circle of Light in December, we all experienced a great shift in consciousness, a transformation for all of us.

There is no way to explain all of the daily miracles we have experienced. God has led us absolutely impeccably through a light-filled awakening of a greater and greater spiritual communion. Fear fell away, as Message by Message, God carefully showed us how to move beyond ego and how to fill our days with gratitude. Then in a very short span of time, these Messages poured forth. Even in all of my sweet and glorious communion with God, I had never experienced anything like this. I was lifted in vibrating waves of golden light.

Each day we would read and absorb the Message. Some of the Messages were answers to our questions, questions that arose as we took in and lived what God had given. Other Messages were poured through me like a rushing river headed outward to humanity. In many of the Messages there is repetition. Yet this repetition is both necessary and purposeful. Every time God repeats something, it is because this is what it takes to make it into our consciousness. You will also find in reading, that every repetition brings with it another new piece, one that requires the repeated concept as its foundation. Another thing to notice is the level at which you read. If you are only in your mind, the repetition may catch your attention. But if you are prayerful, with an open heart, you will be lifted perfectly, step-by-step, concept-by-concept until the shift is born within you.

When the Messages on Sacred Sexuality began, we discovered that as close and loving as we are with each other, we felt embarrassment in discussing the Messages. It was hard to believe, but there it was. When we would discuss what God was showing us, we could hardly use the words. God immediately told us that this embarrassment was a part of the Old World, that for us to believe that sexuality is somehow embarrassing or sinful was to be giving our God- given power away – even to the point of believing that sexual energy must be conquered, transformed or raised up in order to be one who is truly spiritual.

As God revealed the truth in a Message called "The Lie," we were stunned. We committed on the spot to overcome our embarrassment that we could be able to speak easily about the amazing truth of Sacred Sexuality.

So if you find yourself embarrassed about the subject, know that you are not alone! Know too that once you have read these Messages, you will never feel the same again about this topic that is such an intimate and beautiful part of human life. You will find many of your questions answered on these pages in a way that will lift and bless and completely transform anything you thought you knew about LoveMaking.

You will also understand the Divine Masculine and the Divine Feminine, which God often refers to as positive (masculine) and negative (feminine) charges. In using these words to describe these energies, they most closely refer to something more like the electrical poles on a battery and not positive meaning good and negative meaning bad. These "charges" have to do with the spirit and not the body, thus SoulMate pairs can be any gender as long as their spiritual charges are positive and negative.

Every day here at Circle of Light is a miracle. Every single moment we each are able to choose to serve the light, to choose Love, to say "Yes" to Love by speaking the words that are the key to the embodiment of Love for our times: "I want my SoulMate." We offer these Messages with the deepest gratitude and humility and with the continual prayer that we may be only in God's Will, that we may be completely clear and free of self in our receipt and offering of these Messages.

The Messages have completely changed our lives. Even the Messages we could not immediately understand nonetheless blessed us and moved us into greater awareness. We pray for you these same miracles. As you say "Yes" to Love and speak the words "I want my SoulMate;" as your heart opens and Love is revealed, we offer our assistance. For as the coming of Love for this age takes shape in your life, it will completely change your definitions of life and of Love. Then will you too show this path to others, as the proof of God's amazing Love becomes manifest before you—as your SoulMate.

Yael

A note about the word "God": God is beyond words – pure, conscious, all-encompassing Love. God is beyond gender, and yet it includes Divine Masculine and Divine Feminine. Thus do we invite you to use whatever word is comfortable to you as you read these Messages. Know that we honor all words for God. We also embrace all who have embodied God's Love perfectly on Earth.

NOTE FROM THE EDITOR

I met Yael and Doug Powell on July 17th, 2001. God led me right to them through a series of synchronous events. Yael rarely leaves her home but she and Doug had decided very spontaneously to celebrate her birthday at the home of a close friend in Fayetteville. That friend had also graciously agreed to host me, a complete stranger, for a few days, while I explored the Fayetteville, AR area.

As I sat with Yael and Doug that evening, I was fascinated by their obvious living love for each other that pervaded their every word and movement. I learned about Yael's constant pain from a genetic disease of the spine that severely limits her movement, and about Circle of Light, their spiritual center in Eureka Springs. Following dinner Yael read one of the "Messages from God" that have come through her during thirty years of daily meditation. I felt indescribable excitement and upliftment from the extraordinary vibration created and the amazing information of this Message. The topic, completely new to me, was SoulMates.

We quickly recognized ourselves as the ancient Soul Family we are, and spent two bliss-filled days together at Circle of Light, reconnecting, sharing our lives and our spiritual journeys. Our coming together was divinely guided, step-by-step. Yael and Doug showed me fifty hand-written notebooks of Messages from God! I committed myself on the spot to utilizing my writing, editing and organizational skills to help them bring this illuminated and needed material out into the world. I returned to my home in Asheville, N.C., tidied up my life and made plans for a move. Mid-fall by phone, email, and fax we had produced the outline and first drafts of SAY "YES" TO LOVE, God Explains SoulMates. Just before Christmas 2001 I took up residence in my new home at Circle of Light.

After my arrival our "training" began in earnest. The Messages intensified, many with specific personal directives for us. We all experienced a great shift in consciousness that is on-going. Within a few months we had the entire content of *God Unveils SoulMate Love and Sacred Sexuality* (Book II), as well as the third book, *God's Guidance to LightWorkers*.

Life at Circle of Light is a series of marvels. The natural beauty of the lake, mountains and surrounding woods creates the feeling of the New World. Every day Yael meditates several hours, bringing through the amazing teachings from God. The highlight of each day is reading the new Message together. I assist in managing our active wedding business, spend a great deal of time in sorting, compiling and editing Messages, helping with cooking and practical life necessities and tend the organic garden. I have the joyous feeling of knowing I am in the right place at the right time, with my family, doing the tasks for which I have been prepared. I have never been happier! Our commitment as a spiritual family is to bring God's Message of Love forth to our brothers and sisters.

Shanna Mac Lean

...we are talking about
a union of Love
where your heart opens within you so wide
it seems to hurt.
Where Love just pours out from you
to your partner in waves.
Where you are filled with the longing for
your partner to somehow know
how much you love him or her.
Where the definition of your body disappears
as you melt together, becoming one.
Where the climax of your LoveMaking
shoots you out of your body
and expands your being
across the great heavens
and the Dove of Peace settles gently
in your chest.

Where the experience of such Love
is a balm to your spirit
and brings order to your life.
Where you feel that all your days
upon the Earth
and every challenge you have had to
conquer is completely and absolutely worth
it for
One Moment Of Love
such as this.
And where the knowledge of this Love
is so powerful
that it is proof to every part of your being
that I, God, exist
and love you
because I have granted you
such amazing and ecstatic joy.

Part One:
SoulMate Love

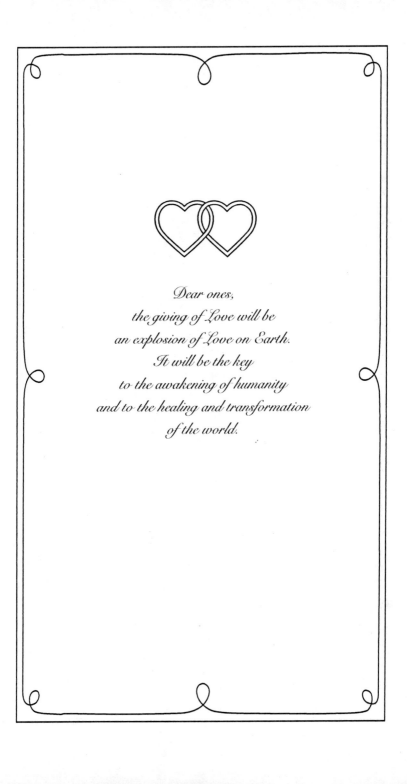

Dear ones,
the giving of Love will be
an explosion of Love on Earth.
It will be the key
to the awakening of humanity
and to the healing and transformation
of the world.

SoulMates:
The Lock and the Key that Together Open the Way to Humanity's Transformation

My beautiful ones, can you picture a cell of My heart? I want you to absorb this question. I want you to stretch to encompass this thought, this wholeness (for "thought" certainly does not contain it!). I want you to do your best, at the highest level possible for you at this time, to understand this. *This is who you are. You are a cell in My heart, the heart of the Creator of All That Is*, The One, the Alpha and Omega, and everything in between — the forces of Light and Love that, moving together, have manifested all life, all worlds, all beauty and filled each and every one of these creations with grace and with the power to transform.

You are at the center of Creation. You, together, exist as cause, not as effect. *You are the beginning of Love. You are the foundation of My being. You are My heart.*

Of course you cannot understand what this means, but you *know.* You know in your own heart, for it is made in My image. You *know* in the awareness that lives within you, in the golden state of grace that is My Love bathing you, and that knowledge is your path Home. You are awakening to that path.

While you cannot understand this with your mind – for your minds are far too limited to hold this — there are keys that will re-awaken this knowledge in you. These keys are living energies, energies that will affect you, bless you and grow you. They are energies most of all that will re-awaken you to what you know. On one level or from one perspective, these things are the most intense and esoteric of all possible human realities. On the other hand, dear ones, they are simple! They are the most basic truths of your existence. As you find them, you will be partaking in a process of awakening that is as natural as a seed sprouting in your garden, nourishing itself, accepting life until it totally transcends what it is in order to become what it is meant to be.

The flower does not think about how to become a plant. It does not struggle with processing a reason to bloom. No. It reaches for the sun as naturally as you awaken each day, and it knows itself when it sees itself bloom. Not before. It has no diagrams of flowering, no one to impress with its brilliance. It only becomes what it is, and so shall you. So shall you – with every bit as much grace. *You are the flower of Creation, the blossoming of My Love that will bring joy and nourishment not only to this world, but to all of Creation as well.*

The first and foremost key in the awakening of humanity is the SoulMate. Do you know how you say that two people fit together like hand and glove? Yes! It is true. It should be two fit together like a lock and key. I tell you that the turning of that key in that lock becomes the opening, the cracking of the seed in the example of our flower. It becomes the moment when what you are gives way to what you will become.

I cannot tell you how profound this is, but your heart will tell you. I cannot tell you because there truly are no words for this miracle of Love. The miracle for which all of your journeys have prepared you — all of your lives, all of your lessons, all of the things you have built and stored over the centuries (millennia!) in the special treasure chest of your

2

highest self, awaiting the moment when all is ready. The moment when you are ready, when your SoulMate is ready, and when humanity is ready. Awaiting the time of the world when everything needed to create the fertile soil of transformation is right there.

This is such a time. This I promise. Let this promise resonate in your heart, dear ones. Let it resonate until you can feel it cracking the shell that surrounds your heart. Let it resonate within you until you are aware of a corresponding resonance — your SoulMate. That resonance is like a foghorn, and it serves such a purpose. It draws you together through the fog of the illusion, even though you cannot see because the fog is too thick. But if you keep listening and keep sending out the call, your SoulMate will be drawn to you just as surely as night is followed by day in this world, for I have laid a course of Love. I have planted the garden of My heart, and what I have planted is you. As I have planted, so shall you. You will also grow a garden of Love within your joined heart – but this is a topic for another time.

So right now you send forth the resonance, the vibration of your true self as deeply and profoundly as you can access your truth. What you can't access you must call on Me to supply. Then you must continue sending forth, sending forth. For if you were a foghorn and you stopped for one moment, what would happen? The boat following your guidance could lose its way. Worse, it could crash into the rocks. *This resonance of heart will become the spiritual signature, the vibrational statement of your truth. It is very important.* Not only will you draw to you your SoulMate. You will also draw all the things that reflect who you are in the world. While this can be positive, it is secondary. *The most important (oh, I can't possibly tell you how important!) is your resonance for your SoulMate.*

3

Now, this resonance of heart must be nourished, checked, tended, cleansed and prepared – just as a garden is prepared for the most precious of flowers. (Yes, there are two metaphors going here – but the imagery is speaking to your subconscious very effectively. It does not matter if it makes sense to the mind.) If you are already in a relationship, you still must carefully establish your heart resonance, for it is this vibrational statement that brings your SoulMate into full manifestation before you. *As your SoulMate is brought into embodiment, it means that your heart is pure enough, loving enough, to have this reflected to you in form.* It is the greatest of blessings. It is absolutely My assurance to you that you are blossoming!

As this beautiful expression of your loving heart comes ever more fully into embodiment, of course an energy exchange takes place. This energy exchange nourishes you and nourishes your SoulMate! The energy/Love which is moved back and forth between you continues to bless and open you both, drawing you closer and closer, and ultimately creating one energy system, as your energy circulates between you. Ultimately, you become One Heart together. The moment you do so, that cell in My heart is "switched on." *That cell in My heart becomes the "light cell" it is meant to be, able to create Love and to move it by Will, together.* Dear ones, what you call light is actively moving Love. It is Love vibrating, Love that is directed, Love given forth. *It is this giving forth, this movement of Love, that is the foundation of Creation. The substance of all things is Love.* The movement that brings Love into form, that makes the flower blossom, is Love directed by Will.

Thus, you began as a cell in My heart, so much a part of Me that there was no real distinction between us. We could not truly relate to each other. If you moved away from Me, the moment you turned back and looked at Me, you automatically came rushing back. You were not co-creators.

You did not have Will of your own. Thus came the journey. "Leaving the Garden" is the perfect description. But now you are coming back! And what is the key to the Garden gate? Knowledge of the SoulMate. What is the key to the bursting open of the seed to become the flower? The lock and key of the SoulMate reunion.

It is difficult to place words upon this. It sounds elementary, yet as you open it will become obvious just how perfect every detail of this journey is, every miracle of transformation of which you are a part. Never let anyone convince you otherwise. Listen deeply within your heart and this truth will be verified.

So whether you are with someone or not, whether you believe that person could possibly be your SoulMate or not, I ask you to trust in Me. Trust Me to set up your soul reunion, to invoke the full memory of the truth of your being, to put forth your heart resonance, the vibrational signature of who you really are. Then make every decision based in this truth. Rejoice in this expectancy, and prepare to be amazed. Even if you can see your SoulMate in the person before you, trust that, as the saying goes, "you ain't seen nothing yet!" Let other things fall easily into place, including the blossoming awareness of the pivotal point in human awakening on which you stand, but keep your focus on your SoulMate.

Do not let the ego in! Do not let the ego engage you in debate about this truth — about whether the SoulMate could be real, about sexuality and whether your SoulMate must be male or female, how they should be, what you require (the worst!), and so on. I tell you again, your SoulMate is the other half of the cell. Together you are one cell of My heart. Without any possibility otherwise, as your heart becomes centered in Love, vibrating in Love, that Love will manifest before you. As above, so below. The exterior is essentially irrelevant.

Yes, there may be certain things you have agreed to do that will influence the "outer package," but as you blossom together everything in the physical world will be drawn into manifestation according to the Love shared between you and pouring through you. Bodies will change! They will heal, glow, become vehicles of light. Circumstances will change, dancing around you like electrons around the nucleus, or planets around a sun. Thus, you can trust that your SoulMate's vibrational resonance will become ever more fully manifested before you, as you manifest the truth of Love that is your being. It is difficult to grasp this in the midst of what you like to call third-dimensional reality, but all of this is changing. And it is changing so beautifully! Oh, dearest ones, please open your hearts! Open to the blessings of this journey of awakening.

Then, as SoulMates come together, an even more magnificent chapter of the dance of life will unfold. Remember how amazing it was the first time you looked into a microscope and saw a whole new world there? Incredible shapes and forms, merging, growing, becoming something new? On the other end of the spectrum, now, this is also happening. On the cosmic level, you are transforming. And as you have always known, the macrocosm and microcosm, and everything between, all reflect each other perfectly. Of course. Because all is one. Creation is all within Me. So what affects one thing affects the whole. This is easy to see. What is more difficult to see, and more exciting, is how perfectly something that happens occurs on every level simultaneously.

This will now be your human course of study in the next few decades. Out of this study will come your full awakening as conscious participants in the communion that is Creation. This beautiful ballet that is life, that is Creation, is being called Sacred Geometry, and humanity is beginning to awaken and become aware of its study. This study will be the platform from which I launch you into your becoming the conscious heart of God. Co-creators. Beings of greatest Love known throughout the All for what you truly are; hidden, with greatest Love and care, in the safe pocket of Time and Space. You are ready. It may not feel like it. When you look around it will seem impossible. But the truth is coded within you. Once humanity accepts the path of the SoulMate the code will be activated. Humankind will know. My heart will become fully conscious.

It is two uniting as one – the cosmic equivalent of the uniting of the sperm and the egg. The moment this occurs, the moment the SoulMates accept the other's existence and the possibility of the SoulMate's manifestation, they begin the move toward each other. The moment of conscious joining turns the key in the lock. At this point the two become one, moving together like a flame, an arrow, penetrating the illusion and traveling easily into the realm of truth. Things that were impossible to understand now open before them.

Then, as the two who are one grow in conscious Will, they begin to create. The two of you will take your place with Me. As I have told you, you will be within Me, yet together you will be awake, separate from Me. Able to relate to Me as co-creators. It already begins, but oh My beloved ones, how it will bless Me as it grows! Yes, you are My great blessing! For in you My Love, My creativity, manifests. You are My surprise, for you will create brand new things born of your spark together, your Love, your awareness, your perspective.

Obviously you cannot co-create with Me while darkness or ego remain in your consciousness. Yet (listen!) the SoulMate path makes it easy to shift out of ego, duality, fear, darkness. This is its greatest gift. For your SoulMate is your choice for Love manifested in front of you. *You have to reach the pure Love and the real trust in Me before you will be able to join with your SoulMate.* Before the key will turn in the lock, your vibrational level must be totally locked into at least the level of the fourth to fifth chakras – the vibrational level of the New World. Then you will be seeing the real world, not the illusion. Then, and only then, will the key turn in the lock and the new consciousness emerge.

At this point, *My call goes out to you, for as My heart leaps in joy, so then does yours. Can you hear the call? Can you remember the truth of Love? Not that it is a possibility, but that it is assured.* I tell you, in this passing age, the question placed before you was Jesus. Christed, he rose as My truth, visible even through the mists of illusion. He was The Way. He was the truth of My Love for that age.

But now you are grown. You are graduating. No longer do you require a teacher to model the truth, in which you must choose to believe. Now you become the truth. And as you become it, as you become Love, Love manifests before you in your life. As I have always told you, all things are embodied. Like attract like. If you are in Love (meaning living in the truth of your heart), that Love will manifest before you. And when it does, you know that the key is in your hand (or rather, the key is your heart).

These are the basics. Now we will begin the advanced. The blessing of the union – yes! *The opening of the flower of life; the truth of the Sacred Geometry — that Love sings itself into being on every level and fills the world with light. And all the places that were void, the places where Love was not, are filled through your intention, and everything returns to perfection.* Every body is healed. Once the SoulMate is embraced, every heart becomes the living flower echoing My heart and bringing My heart into the world! Through that flower of the human heart, all things are connected in Love. (Ah, if you thought the "lotus" of the crown chakra was something, wait until you see the joined SoulMate heart!)

8

It will all change in an instant. Faster than the speed of thought is the truth of Love. I will guide you. I will tenderly and gently release your grip on the illusion. I will, with the greatest respect, prepare your heart for opening. I will fertilize the ground of your consciousness with My promises of what is to come. And I will adorn the heavens with your beauty. As you emerge, I will say to all who will listen:

Did you have a doubt? Did you doubt that what I held within My own heart could be true? Did you doubt that real Love would be reflected, magnified, expanded, in the truth of the SoulMate heart? And could you see that nothing could stand against the force of My light, even as it is reflected by two beings who are SoulMates?

I bid you welcome, for I Am The One, and the awakening of My heart is producing the greatest light ever yet known. To the farthest reaches of Creation comes the shining report that I Am The One and that My living heart is growing, in just the way we planned. Oh, there can be no rigid parameters when it comes to My heart's awakening, for it is the answer to My intention, My call, that humanity have Will -- that they, being My progeny, can also create as I can. As they grow into their truth, the truth of their Love, I ask that All Within Me, I Who Am the All in All, embrace them with Love. For they can only stand before Me with their own Will, and thus, as always, will they teach Me about Myself.

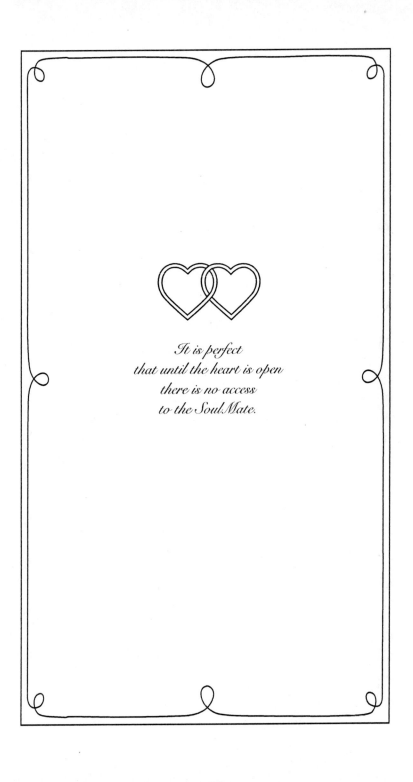

*It is perfect
that until the heart is open
there is no access
to the Soul Mate.*

Opening to Your SoulMate Now Becomes the Most Important Spiritual Task in the World

My blessed, beloved and precious humanity, I pour the golden light of your awakening upon you. I gently lift your vision. I wash the sleep from your eyes. And I place My hand upon your heart and say to you: "Awaken to the manifestation of Love in your life. Awaken to your SoulMate."

In this, I supersede even the Christ, who is to you the pouring forth of My living Love in form. I say to you that in this age this Love of Mine is even closer. It is closer than the one who came to wear the mantle of Christ as proof of your place in My heart! Closer than anything except perhaps this body you are wearing. It is close enough that you can see your magnificence right before you. Close enough that you can see My hand upon your heart, for My hand upon your heart will manifest now as the greatest of all My gifts to you — the presence of your SoulMate.

Opening to your SoulMate now becomes the most important spiritual task in the world, for together you can know me perfectly as I stand before you as your perfect Love.

Oh, My beloved humanity! Would that you could know how much I love you, how deeply I know you, how perfectly you are created! In this age I bring you more than "My only begotten son." In this age I give you the precious mirror of your own divine Love—your SoulMate. Not as a figure rising above you as an example. Rather, as the complete experience of total and personal immersion in perfect divine Love.

Through this Love I now promise you the ability to truly know yourself, to know yourself as Love in form, as Love in action, as My Love, as My child in the world. Closer than any and every example ever given to you yet, this New Age of Love, the Millennium of the Awakening, is the time when you at last can experience who you really are. In creating you I knew that My greatest wish was a complimentary consciousness with which to share My Love and glory. Knowing this, dearest ones, I created you already including this greatest gift—that complementary consciousness. You would have perfect Love, and you would know through your SoulMate, the truth of our relationship.

What you are to Me—the surprise of Love that expands Me, the consciousness that reflects Me and the living form of My great out-going Love, this your SoulMate is to you. As you are a piece of My living heart, filled with the essence of the Love that I am, so is your SoulMate a piece of your own heart, manifested before you, as you are manifested before Me. As you grow, so am I able to see My Love blossom in you. As you grow, so will you see your SoulMate manifesting ever more clearly before you.

Most important of all, as I love you, and in My Love give to you all of Me, so too, as you open in Love with your SoulMate will the two of you together give back to Me. As you know Love in its amazing beauty, in its power and in its sweetness, so will your joined heart sing in gratitude and in the giving forth of Love. You will receive the fullness of My Love together and you will give forth to All That Is. And in this giving, in your Love you will open your hearts to the joy of our communion. Then will the circle be complete. Love will then flow perfectly through all Creation, and Creation will become a living being—out of which you will create new worlds.

It is difficult as always to explain but I attempt to pour this vision into your minds and hearts because as you grasp it, you will rise up into the truth of your being. *SoulMates are — together, individually — hearts within My heart, ready to nourish your own Creation while lovingly sharing the entirety of Mine.* Thus I stretch you to the vision of how vast you are, how beautiful, how deeply your awareness grows, and of the power of reunion with your SoulMate.

I am offering you the personal experience of My Love. Closer than the story of Jesus, I tell you the story of your SoulMate. For understanding this — the existence of the rest of your heart — you will at last understand many things in your lives. You will understand the inner nudgings. You will understand the whisper in your consciousness and the longing in your heart. All you have to do is move away from your ego and into your heart. Your SoulMate will then come to you.

Not only are Twin Flames, or SoulMates, the personal experience of My Love for you every moment of every day. They are the affirmation of the law of Love. *If Love is what is in you, then Love will appear before you.* Thus to open to your SoulMate (in truth, to see what is already there), you need only move completely into your heart.

Not only is your SoulMate your experience of Love in form—My Love for you and proof of your true nature. Your SoulMate is the consciousness that will show you who you are. Thus will you immediately begin to open to the fullness of your creative ability and the great breadth of your awareness as you have another consciousness with which to share your divinity.

Yet there is more! Not only is your SoulMate the assurance of My great Love for you — that I would give you such a gift — but when you are reunited, a piece of My heart is healed. Your Love in your new conscious individuality as awakened humans activates the piece of My heart that you are—giving it new and greater consciousness! Thus I am expanded in My Love as well! Yes, it is true. I am all Love, and yet you will make Me even more.

And there is even more than this! You know, of course, that everything is consciousness. "As above, so below" is the truth of consciousness on every level of Creation. Thus are all things embodied and fully conscious, whether the embodiment is physical or the greatest cosmic light. As SoulMates awaken, you become living hearts of Creation. You are a heart in your own right, while you are a conscious cell in Mine. You become the center of a new universe. Beating together, you pour forth Love and everything in your consciousness comes alive. You become the creator to the universe that you form! Thus you are the surprise to Me also, bringing forth new worlds of beauty and complexity and glory. Are you beginning to sense the magnitude of this? (And, of course, there is very great need for you to have control of your consciousness, since all that you create in your consciousness is imbued with life through your Love.)

Last, but certainly not least! As you become the living heart, the two of you together, you have the ability to open this heart that you are to Me. You can open it and allow Me to pour My Love through you in order to lift your creation into the greatest harmony — into alignment with My Creation, with All That Is. The moment you do this you fully connect yourselves to All That Is, to Me, to the great Love and to the great plan for All That Is.

Oh, My beloved ones, it is here, as you become the living heart in alignment with My greater heart that you are complete. Home. A part of the unbroken circle, the truth of Love. Truly Home. Heart within My heart, you will be ever uplifted in unimaginable joy. Here there truly is no possibility of communicating this to you in any mental images. I invite you to come into your heart and ask, and I will show you as much as you can hold of this greater truth.

All the "levels" of heaven, all the hierarchies of evolution, are the many ways people have chosen to come Home. They are not necessary. There is no climb, dear ones. There are no initiations you must take. It is all, in truth, totally a matter of consciousness. You are co-creators. What you believe is what you experience. Thus, if you know the truth, with all your heart and all your consciousness, you can find Home in your SoulMate's eyes and you can accomplish the "journey" in the communion of your hearts. Your SoulMate is the one criterion, for he or she already exists as part of you.

Thus if you are not seeing him or her, you are caught in the illusion, for in truth, he is there. Obviously, then, you must open your heart enough to see the true world, the world of Love and unity, the world in which you can see what you have always had.

Because together you are the union of the forces of Creation, you will bring these energies back into presence in the world. Using them, letting the Divine Masculine and Divine Feminine return to Earth in you, you can and must change everything. In your Love you will lift the Earth and all the beauty upon and within it back into the vibration of Love. Being a heart of Creation, My beloved SoulMates, you can easily do this consciously. So you see that this is the way you will lift up the Earth and bring all life back into the reality of Love, the reality of abundance, of plenty, of truth and perfection.

That, dear ones, is how you can "get there from here!" That is how you can save the Earth. That is how you can return all her verdant life to her, including those you believe to be extinct. In the truth of Love, everything is perfect, as all of Nature has revealed to you, along with your precious animals. Everything exists in wholeness and beauty.

So just as you are learning that you can see relationship through the ego or the heart, so too can you see the world either way. If you are in your ego, you could see your precious SoulMate only as someone who might hurt you. You could see your world as filled with competition, jealousy and striving, not to mention "bad things" happening continually. Yet if you are in your heart, you see your SoulMate, and you link to a truth that gets bigger and bigger. You see the Divine Plan in which you have come together over eons of time to awaken huge numbers of people—that your own awakening would do the most good. You will see the amazing Love between you that has no beginning and no end. And every time you look with your heart at your true Love, you see more and more ways that together you can be a blessing to the world and to humanity.

Just so can you also see the Earth and all upon it as a doomed planet of limited resources and terrible divisiveness. Or you can see the world through your heart, as a place of the most beautiful unity. If you do either from the position of union with your SoulMate, you will create it.

Obviously, to see your SoulMate, to see the other half of you, your Twin Flame (which is the more accurate term), you must be seeing with your heart. Thus when together will you easily see the world as Love as well. Doing this, dear ones, you can quickly change the world, for SoulMates together are My Love in form. Add Will to divine Love, and creation occurs. Thus *I ask you to know that you can easily manifest the New World consciously with your SoulMate.*

Right now in human awakening there is nothing more important than opening to the SoulMate. I can

16

promise you that as soon as you experience the Love of your SoulMate you will see everything else correctly. You will understand. To put this "Biblically," to come back to the Garden, Adam and Eve must find each other, for that Garden is made for two, Adam and Eve, you and your SoulMate, because that is how you already exist! Your SoulMate is part of you. This is a FACT. Twin Flames. Two halves of one whole. Two sides of One heart. Two reflections of One consciousness.

The forgetting time is OVER. To find your individuality, you have taken many forms, separated from the truth so you would believe you were alone. This was an important part of a very important plan. But at the end of the "involution," of your journey of individuality, we agreed that you would know it was time to turn back toward Me — when you were reunited with your SoulMate. If you ask yourself, deeply, you will remember this is true. Thus, I call you to remember. It is time for the journey of awakening.

Dear ones, in truth every bit of this journey is about what you agreed to believe. Please read this again. Do you remember? Think about this! You could not "forget" who you are unless you chose it. God cannot forget. But we knew, together, that you could not exist individually unless you could journey far enough away that you could "get out of My orbit" so to speak. You had to forget who you were long enough to build an identity that would prevent you from flying right back into the vastness that I Am.

We have accomplished this! Oh, is this not the greatest reason to rejoice? Now, My beloved ones, all you have to do is remember. There is nothing else. There are no "levels" you must climb, no evolutions through various dimensions, unless you believe there are. All of those things are for those who are still forgetting. All those "heavenly realms," all those higher and higher levels of learning are created for those who are still partly sleeping. You do not need to do this. *All you must do is remember, and the agreed upon method for you to remember everything is to look into the eyes and heart of your SoulMate.*

I promise you that this is true. This is the only "path" you need, and, it can happen in an instant — the full recovery of your complete identity as the joined heart of divine Twin Flames. In that instant, you can reclaim your co-creatorship with Me.

Thus, this SoulMate information is the most important information in the world. Please, do all you can, every one of you, to disseminate it. Share these messages in every language. And for you who say "yes," who remember and open your heart, share your experience as your SoulMate reappears.

In the last age, Jesus wore the mantle of My Love in form. Now you are all ready to experience this. He said: "Blessed are those who do not see, but believe anyway." Now I say: "Blessed are those who believe, for they will see Love." Standing before them. Their SoulMate.

Dear ones, in this age, Love is come to live in you, and living in you it must manifest in your life. This is the law of Creation. Like attracts like. All energies are embodied. Thus, your own Love, the truth of who you are must, by this law, be embodied in your life.

The only reason people cannot see their SoulMate is that they do not have real Love within them. Therefore, they see only the vibration of the "false" world, the world of separation and ego. So each of you must help others to choose to live from the heart, for then it is the law that their SoulMate will appear. If any who want their SoulMate are not finding him or her, then they are still living in the ego, whether or not they will admit it. *It takes effort to shift into the heart in the face of the mass consciousness.*

Thus do you who know have your "work cut out for you" in showing others how to make this shift. But, oh the rewards! Not only for those who open up, who change their lives, but also for you who are awake. For it is far more true than you can possibly conceive, that "in giving you receive." If you did nothing else but unselfishly give to others, your transcendence would be assured. Energy is a moving thing. In order to receive its benefits, it must be moving through, heading outward. Thus will it ever be alive, just as the heart must move the blood through your body in order for you to be alive. As your blood feeds the body's cells, so does giving of Love feed your spiritual bodies. It must not ever cease. The more Love given, the more light released, the more that flows through your own system.

The signal of your homecoming is the reunion with your SoulMate. Yet, to do so, you must remember that you are Love, that you can "see" with the heart, that there is a choice between ego and Love. Each and every human being has a seed of remembrance within. *Your work as you are awakening is to also seek every way to bring forth this memory in every human being.* Never be discouraged. Always remember that the shift can be instantaneous. Truly. All it takes is that one jogged memory, the "aha" experience, and all it takes for those of you who are with your SoulMates to lift yourselves back into the fullness of our relationship is just as simple. One moment of complete union with your SoulMate can do it, for truly you are as you believe. I will keep reminding you of this so you can release your limiting visions.

You are creating all of it, My beloved ones — by our agreement, yes, but also by your creative ability. *You have imagined this world of your separation, and all that is a*

19

part of this world is the symbolic language of what you are currently believing. Believe in your Love! We have made this easy because your Love will manifest before you. Then, moment by precious moment, you will be able to see whether you are recognizing your true nature. How? By observing your Love for your SoulMate.

Dear ones, believe in Love as the truth of your being and believe in its manifestation as your SoulMate. Watch carefully. If your SoulMate has not manifested and you call for them, note that from that moment they are with you, waiting for you to see them. *If you are with someone, they can come through that person.* If you don't see any way then you are limiting your capability, for this world is completely an illusion. The fact that you are with someone with whom "there is no way" says something about you, not them. You must look at it this way! You must acknowledge that this is your dream. *Why would you have dreamed this, that in the life where you are waking up, you have chosen to be with someone who is not? Be rigorously honest. Choose to love them unconditionally and to see them as a potential vehicle for your SoulMate.* Then take action.

In most cases where a person waking is with someone asleep, there is a deep resistance to "rocking the boat." There is a need for security, a lack of belief that no matter what, your good will come to you. However, it is the unwillingness to "shatter the comfort zone" that is often the issue. Not always—remember this is just an example to get you thinking.

If this were what you discovered after deep examination, plus calling Me to assist you to see, you would need to go to your mate. You would need to tell them that you believe they are your SoulMate, but that you have reached a point where you must share it consciously. Explain what that means. Explain, explain, explain. Explain that you know you will leave the relationship if it is not expressed, but keep reiterating that you firmly believe they are able to be your SoulMate. *You must be prepared to be amazed.*

If you are not prepared to be amazed, you are in your ego. If you feel there is "too much water under the bridge" (please listen), you are not in your heart, you are in your ego. I now ask you, those in such a situation, to be sure you are living in your heart and that you have been rigorously honest with yourself and lovingly positive yet honest with them. If you are absolutely sure you have completely moved from ego to heart and you look, you will begin to see your SoulMate. Yes, in them, in that person you have JUDGED as unable or unworthy. I guarantee you that *your SoulMate is standing right there, waiting to "overshadow" your partner.*

I want to tell you, all of you, to expect miracles. Oh, the time of the world is changed, for in your heart you will see the truth. If you are waking, I can promise you there is a reason you are with your partner. *You will soon hear many stories of people who had almost given up in despair, who shifted to the heart and found their SoulMate there.*

If you have completely and honestly shifted to your heart as your regular level of perception (please pay attention here) and you have been deeply loving yet truthful, before you leave a relationship, be sure you have clear signs from Me. For many times the opening of the person you are with is one of the major pre-incarnation commitments of service you made. However, it is possible for someone to be so entrenched in ego as to be lost. But it would be very unusual that you, an awakening one, would be with them. But not impossible. Thus, I ask you to step carefully. For it might be easier for you to see your SoulMate through someone new because you believe you could, but you might discover you had left behind some unfinished business in you.

I say these things to you because, dear ones, the veils are thinning. Help is all around you. The truth is ever more visibly in front of you—that *your world is about what you believe. Remember this and it can change in an instant.*

I am not saying that it is never correct to leave someone to go in search of your SoulMate. I am saying that the truth is a matter of choosing to see Love. Just be sure you have truly done so. Your life can certainly be changed by moving what you believe is outside of yourself, and right now this seems more real to you. But it can also be changed just as fully by moving what is inside of you.

In our examination of the awakening of Love, the reunion of SoulMates, I will present this from every different viewpoint so that every one of you can find yourselves in these words and can come to the deepest reflection of Love possible in the shortest amount of time. For *the awakening is upon you and your SoulMate is the most important piece.*

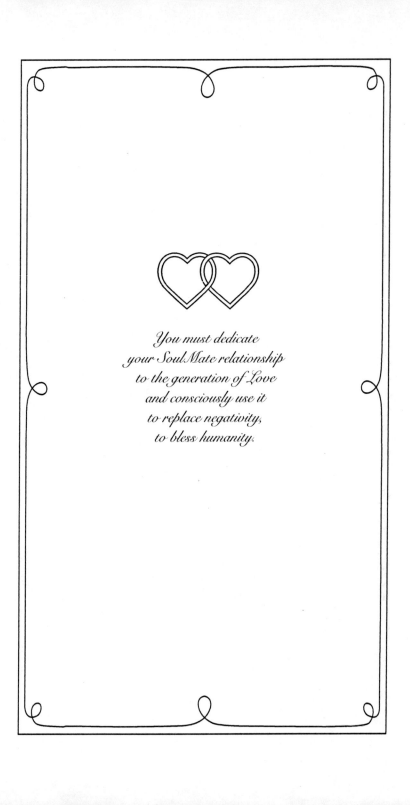

*You must dedicate
your SoulMate relationship
to the generation of Love
and consciously use it
to replace negativity,
to bless humanity.*

When SoulMates Return into Conscious Relationship, The Healing of Love Is Complete

I am here with you, pouring My light down. Within My heart lies the perfection of Love, every answer to every question and an ever-reaching energy of Love seeking to bless everything with Love. In My heart, in the perfection of every cell, lies the blueprint of Love that is the truth of humankind. In every cell in My heart there is balance — the two beings that are one Love. The two mirrors, reflecting and thus balancing the energy of Love, which is the energy that sustains all of creation.

Thus, if you are the physical cells of My heart, you are the movement of all Love into form. You cannot understand the truth of this yet, but I ask you to stretch to encompass this.

When SoulMates return into conscious relationship, the healing of Love is complete. Everything that has moved away from Love is now called back by the fact of the reunion of SoulMates. Dear ones, when you say "yes," when your SoulMate is with you, you become the proof of the healing of Love.

When you have grown in your Love for your SoulMate, when your heart is reflecting only the purest Love, then, in union, you become the heart of your own creation. Two SoulMates together are a force of creation. You are the seed of a universe of your own creating. The power of the Love flowing through you is the power of life, the substance of

Creation. Together you will begin to love your creation. You will begin to nourish your universe. Thus will I be expanded.

Right now you are just in the very beginning. You are barely awakened to the truth of SoulMate Love. But I must inform you even now that you are a force of creation, because your first creation is to be the New World.

My beloved humanity, it is time for the arrival of Love. It is time now for the coming of Christ, and Christ is the living form of My Love. The birth of the Christ that is coming is within you. What you must grow into is that My Love contains both the masculine and the feminine in order to be a force of movement, in order to create. In order to spark life into its truth, to lead you to the awakening, I am awakening both the Divine Feminine and Divine Masculine within you. In other words, it is time for you to live and understand your truth.

As you say "yes," My beautiful ones, and you open your world to the truth of Love, your SoulMate will manifest with you quickly. You then can begin the healing of the world. This will be your first step. As you fully embody the two energies, you will move into your larger creation, where you become the force that anchors the New World of humanity, where everything is experienced at the level of Love. Then you become another heart of creation, together moving forth to fully co-create.

It is the time of the return of the embodiment of Christ as both the Divine Masculine and the Divine Feminine. It is true that the Divine Masculine, or Christed Masculine, has been present in humanity's consciousness since Jesus anchored it here. But it is not alive in humanity, not embodied yet in the heart of every man. Thus, to the men, I call to you. I remind you of your truth. I call to those who understand that you must make way for the advent of the Divine Feminine, which is coming now. *The completion of the Christ upon the Earth is the birth now of the Divine Feminine. The completion of humanity is the reunion of the whole of Christ, the Divine Masculine and the Divine Feminine.*

As you allow the truth of Love to live in you, you will become, together, this reunion. In you will the balance of Love be revealed. *This reunion is the most important thing that will occur, for as SoulMates come together, the truth of Love will be anchored in the world.* Every SoulMate couple will be the receptors of these divine energies. The perfection of creation, of nurturance and Will, will be embodied.

The moment two SoulMates are rejoined, together they become an anchor for perfect, balanced Love as a force of creation. Automatically Love will pour through them so that Love can be fully present in the world. Christ returns to Earth. Christ is born as the couple, the moment their hearts are linked, and from that moment, the couple will be used to draw into existence the perfect expression of Love in the world.

Dear ones, the "yes" in your heart that puts you on the path of reunion with your SoulMate is the single greatest service you can do for the world and for My precious humanity. Plus, this "yes" in your heart will re-establish divine order in your own life effortlessly. Why? Because it places Love first above everything. When Love is the first and most important thing in your life, everything else will come into perfect alignment, because Love is the highest truth of creation. This wholeness of Love, this return to perfection will also bring you the greatest joy. This I promise you. Whatever your ego believes to the contrary, the reunion of Love is the proof of who you are. It speaks to the depth of your being. You are designed to experience the truth of your divinity through the reflection of your SoulMate's consciousness.

Divine Feminine and Divine Masculine are the forces of movement by which I create All That Is. Thus, everywhere in Creation these two forces exist. Regardless of the myriad interpretations placed on this, it is a truth of Creation. All life everywhere is moved by these two forces, even when they do not overtly manifest. Thus, there is a call in the depth of your being that reaches for your reunion with your SoulMate. Though you may as yet be unable to fully grasp the how or even the why of this, if you say "yes" to Love, you will know its truth when it embodies itself before you. You will know the connection, Divine Masculine and Divine Feminine. Without words, even without mental understanding, you will be sure that together you and your SoulMate are right for the world. You will know that the Love that pours through you is a healing force and a force of creation. For Love speaks the language that is beyond the scope of words.

To those who are still afraid of Love, I whisper that one moment of true Love will turn your fears to dust. One moment, dear ones, and you will know without a shadow of a doubt, that fear of Love has been the greatest lie perpetrated upon you. Fear of Love is the trick of the anti-Christ. But that time is now over. All of Creation is now moving in harmony to support the emergence of Love in humanity. All that is real in Creation, that is. The lie is not real! It is a shadow play. It is finger puppets on the walls of the ego at midnight. But the light is coming on! So brilliantly, with such radiance, that shadows cannot remain.

The only way now that anyone on Earth can remain in the darkness is by choosing to turn his or her face away from Me. Anything else will fall away. So very quickly now the choice for Love will become obvious. As it does, true Love will incarnate here! Let Me say this again. *True Love will incarnate on Earth.* As it does, the Love within Nature will come to embrace you. The Love of the angels will illuminate you. Your SoulMate will reclaim you so that Love is fully incarnate on Earth – so that Christ returns.

All of this Love will easily illumine you. It will pour its gentle light on everything. And guess what will happen? The shadows will fade, the lies will disappear and you will be living in the New World. *The Golden Age is the truth of Love manifested in the world.* It is the reversal of the mistake that you made in the Garden. For there you chose to believe in good *and* evil, and thus you turned your lovely eyes away from their constant focus on My face, My Love, the awareness of your truth.

Now as you choose to see only Love, you will turn back again. The shadow dance will fade, because it is your belief in it that has sustained it. You will know that you are Love incarnate. You are Christ, the truth of My Love, and the Love within you will draw all Love to you and bring the world back to the truth.

In Love you will see what really is, not what the shadows had painted for you, and as you see Love, the power of that sight brings forth that truth in everything. Thus will the Earth be returned to splendor. Thus will the desert of your wanderings be replaced by the truth of Love that has always existed, even while you believed in destruction and death.

You do not even need to understand "dimensions," or what is happening as you are raised up in Love. *What you do need to understand is that every couple that is living in Love is the conduit through which Love is poured into the world. It is contagious!* The more people who experience Love, the more people will believe in it, because the Love pouring into the world through the new incarnation of Christ, will clear away the fog of the lower vibrations. The shadows, the lie, will clear all around them. So when others come near a loving couple, in their presence they will be able to see! The light will be bright enough that all who come near them will be bathed in it. And if even for a moment the fog disappears, each person who has such an experience is forever changed.

I will tell you again that I am Love. As I moved upon the void, I became the two who are one – the blessed womb and the Will to create something within that womb. Thus was Creation born. Thus will it always be. I am ready to have you back, that My longing for companionship be fulfilled, for you are My heart. You are My progeny. In you the truth of Love is evident. As you awaken you will understand how each cell within My heart becomes a heart itself. As you embrace your destiny, you will see yourselves, the whole of Christ, the movement of My Love. You will know then how to begin to beat as one together, the masculine and feminine— the womb and the spark of life within it.

You will comprehend your truth as the embodiment of the Twin Rays of Love as they pour forth from Me. Knowing this, you will heal and raise the Earth that has so lovingly nurtured you. You will illuminate all of humanity, that they too can turn back to the light, step into the truth, say "yes" to Love, and embody the Christ as both the masculine and the feminine that I am as Creation. Then, when the light has spread easily upon the Earth, you will begin to co-create together in ever-greater ways. You will bless new worlds and shape new galaxies. You will understand how you expand Me and surprise Me as you embrace the truth of Love. And the days when you played in shadows will become a distant memory.

Thus do I show you the deepest truth of Love. I challenge you to test it. Choose to believe only in Love, to turn back to the light of My presence. In what will you place your faith? The truth is now everywhere around you. The increasing activity of fear in the world will begin to make the choice obvious, for quickly people will realize that they cannot live like that. Those who are following the media frenzy and allowing fear to consume them will quickly realize it is impossible to bear indefinitely. By exposure to this intensity of the shadow dance, there will come a collective realization that it cannot sustain life. There is no nourishment of soul or spirit in the shadows.

Even if My beloved ones follow the fear until they collapse, then they will have to let go, for they will not have the energy to sustain themselves. At that moment, the light will be there. The angels will surround them. *It is My will that no one will be lost. Please remember this. I will not leave a cell of My heart in darkness!* It would not make sense, would it? Of course not. So knowing this eliminates the possibility of judgment. You are all my progeny. My heart. So none will be left behind.

Therefore, I ask of you who can hear Me, your complete dedication to allowing Me to pour My Love through you. *Please, find your SoulMate quickly that you can be the incarnated Christ, that I may pour My Love into the world through you.* You are the bridge upon which the others will come, for you will make the light accessible. You will make the Love available. As you know, I cannot pour forth too much light without burning those who have been sitting in the shadows – those whose eyes are not yet adjusted to the light. But you can deliver it perfectly because you can modulate it to the current atmosphere — simply by opening your heart.

Oh, let me pour My Love through you. Open yourselves completely. Trust the truth of Love. If you open genuinely, I promise you it will appear before you as your SoulMate. But you must face the light. You must be willing to see him or her. You must be ready to stand against the ego. At first, it will fight, for it is vibrationally very close to the physical. Both the body and the ego have a survival mechanism programmed in by fear. But with every choice for Love, your face is turned more and more fully to My light. It will begin to warm you, and the color of your world will change. Gone will be the dreary grays, the empty moments of isolation. In their place Love will appear, as all Creation begins to be revealed in the light.

For those of you who are living ever more fully in Love, please be sure to dedicate your light to the illumination of your brothers, the awakening of your sisters, for in giving Love you receive Love, and lift your own life closer to Me. Don't forget the power of a loving word, a thought, especially a prayer. And always remember the moment that you understood, the moment that you realized you could open your heart, the moment you awakened to the power of the choice of choosing Love over ego, Love over fear, light over darkness.

Be sure that all with whom you come in contact have this information. Find a way to deliver it, to translate it. Find a way to use the gift of your Love to illuminate them. None come to you by accident. Ever. And *I plant you who are awake, dear ones, deeply into the world, that you will be the conduit there, at every level, through which I can pour My Love.* Please be sure delivery is successful. Ask, and I will show you. If you cannot accomplish it on the conscious level, be sure to deliver it as energy.

Last, but certainly not least, I especially thank those of you who have volunteered to serve as the transformers. You,

My LightWorkers, have given Me the greatest gift — greater than I ever hoped. You have understood My deepest Love and offered your assistance in lifting up all of My beloved ones into Love that I may hold every cherished human heart right away. You have offered to do more than your share, to bring light quickly into the shadows so all My precious ones can see. I cannot even begin to speak in words the magnitude of your gift. Though I longed for all of you, I expected to have to separate those who could not say "yes" to Love now. But you, being on Earth, you can allow My Love to work through you to light every life, to consume every shadow. Thus I thank you again for the LightWorkers' decision, out of which has come an outpouring of response from beings throughout Creation who have rushed forward to assist you.

In this decision you have become as suns, allowing the light to pour through you into every corner of this reality. What this means is that as part of this work, you must turn back around to face the shadows, that you may illuminate them. Thus all of you whose lives would normally be only Love and joy and light, are still touching the illusion, still seeing the shadows, still exposed to the lie. It is not an easy path, but how it proves to Me that all I have known is true. That you have stood the test and taken free will and molded it to the design of your heart. Those who have long scoffed at the plan of free will stand in awe, and Creation expands in gratitude.

As you manifest Love before you as your SoulMate, it will become more obvious to you that these shadows are not yours. I will begin to show you how to move fully into your transformative power as I show you how to live multi-dimensionally. It will become easier to stay in the consciousness of Love as you walk straight into the deepest shadow in order to bring forth the light.

Oh, dear ones, light lives right here, in the midst of the darkness. Love is fully present even in the midst of ego. The New World is here, woven into the fabric of this reality. Soon you will really see it, for your perception will switch. What you thought was real will fade to the background. What you hoped for and longed for will move quickly to the fore and will become the basis of your reality. Where the two meet, you will be able to see and you will then be able to keep adding light until the background is free of all shadows and Love is the only reality.

I will continue to place the vision before you of this expansion of Love, of the delivery of light, until you will find it hard to remember that you ever believed in anything else.

I am with you. Welcome to the world of Love.

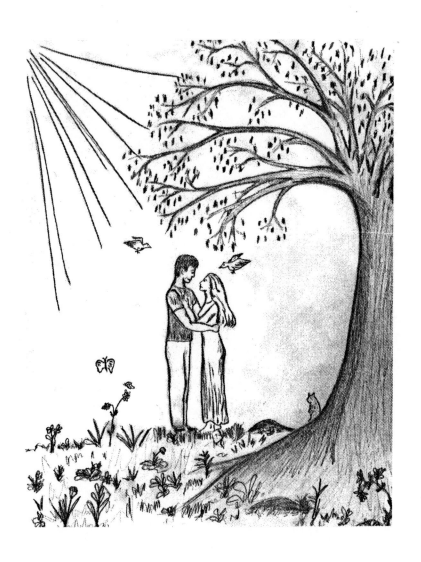

Living in the New World

SoulMates Bring About the Awakening of Humanity and the Earth

It is time for the reunion of SoulMates. As you take the hand of your Twin Flame, as you unite your hearts together into one in the promise to take your Love together as high as it will go, you will participate in the greatest alchemy. You will participate in the return of humanity to its divine state — the transformation of the "base metal" of normal human consciousness into the true gold of your divine destiny.

When you join your hearts, your lives and your destiny, you will follow your divine nature back home to Me. You will follow the two great forces out of which Creation comes – the Divine Masculine and the Divine Feminine – straight up until you meet Me, the All, the essence of Creation, the living Love from which you are made. This is the goal of Sacred Sexuality.

Having followed your true essence back beyond the "First Split," you will be bathed in the perfection of Love, All That Is, all that ever shall be, all Love contained, still waiting. Then, by the power of your essential natures, joined together in perfect Love, you will move upon the "Deep." Together you will retrace the path that I took – the Womb of Love sparked by the Will of God that moves forth into new life. From this moment, this moment of perfect joined communion with Me, by your combined Love and Will — you, the SoulMates, will claim your heritage and you will bring forth a new creation.

Oh, it is so difficult to bring this into words. But can you feel it? Can you sense and know the truth of this? *Together, in sacred union, you fully become the cosmic forces of Divine Feminine and Divine Masculine.* By those very forces, powered by the upliftment of your sexual union (the orgasm), you will retrace your essence upward, up, up, opening along the way into the full experience of pure energy (pure masculine or pure feminine). You will then move beyond all manifestation into pure essence, until you rejoin the All, the sacred pool of My Love, undivided —the Deep that existed before the movement that is Creation. Then, returning, you will know of what you are made. *You will know pure Love.* Pure Love that has no imprint upon it, not even that of Divine Masculine or Divine Feminine. You will know pure Love, before the idea in Me that caused the movement of My Will upon the deep ocean of My being, which is Love.

Knowing this Love you will never be the same. Knowing this Love, you will forever be aware of that Love within everything. You will never be fooled again. You will never be fooled into believing someone's illusion, their personality, and the picture they are attempting to portray. Instead, in everything and everyone, you will see perfect Love, and you will always be participating in right action and right relationship. The moment you see Love behind every facade (listen, as I remind you of this), you affirm that Love is every person's true reality, and thus you will bring it about. You will draw out the true Love in everyone you meet.

Yet this is only one small piece. Once you have traveled the great rays of Creation with your SoulMate, then together you know exactly how to create. You understand the substance of Creation, the perfect unmoving Love. You also understand deeply the real nature of *your* being. You know intimately the power and the presence of your Divine Masculinity. Your Divine Femininity. Not some cultural explanation. Not some distressed psychological touchstone based on countless lifetimes of human family. No. *You will at last understand what it means to be Divinely Masculine, Divinely Feminine, and to be united with your Twin Flame, the other half of your being, as I made you.*

You will have become the forces of Creation. Knowing this, as you look into each other's eyes, heart, and soul, *you will share a complete, consuming desire to bring this gift to the rest of humanity.* Not only because you have experienced something amazing – but also because you will know it is every person's divine destiny. Having moved beyond this tiny pocket of Time, you will understand that it is already here.

This, dear ones, is Sacred Sexuality. If these words do not convey it adequately to you then I ask that you hold these pages and open your heart and allow Me to take you to the awareness of such an experience.

This is the transformation of the world. Why? Because you are the world. Oh, you are far bigger than you realize. How could you not be, for you are My creation! The return to you of your conscious relationship with your SoulMate means you are ready. It would not happen otherwise. It means you have said "yes" to Love. It means that you have chosen to leave the ego behind, that you have become willing to see only Love, to be only Love, to live only Love, and to thus invite the experience of your divinity, your divine nature.

Saying "yes" to Love means your awakening to who you are, which is Love. Awakening to who I am, which is Love. And awakening thus to the full spectrum of your beings – the HUGE reality of Love as it has moved forth by My Will into billions of forms, woven into a tapestry of worlds and dimensions, and the glowing and continual emergence of Love in relationship that is Creation.

The very first Love in relationship was the movement of the parts of Myself within My being – the spark, the idea, and the Will to bring something forth. This first movement was, and still is, the relationship of Divine Masculine and Divine Feminine. Reflecting this, you are the cells within My very heart – the pieces of Love born within the All of Love in order that Love be made manifest.

Knowing this is who you are, I ask you to see that you are the movement of Love brought forth into form. You. Dear ones, this will be difficult for you to comprehend yet, but I will place this before you just to entertain it, if even momentarily, as a possibility. Then you can let it go again, but I want the seed planted firmly within you, the seed of this truth. *You are co-creators of great cosmic proportion, for you are My Heart. You are the cells of the heart of God. Within you is all of the universe of form reaching from the huge form of My very heart all the way down to these little bodies.* It is all within you. As All That Is exists within Me, All That Is the form of Love exists within you. You are My heart and therefore you reach, together as SoulMates, to encompass all worlds of awakening Love.

Right now you are dreaming that you are tiny little beings trapped on one world surrounded by life, disconnected from Love. But as you remember, this reality of which I speak will simply be uplifted within you until its truth is all that is revealed. Then you will see that in your collective hearts, you are nourishing the Earth and its heavens, reaching all the way back to the great cosmic moment of the "First Split" when I became the idea that moved upon the Love of My being.

When you grasp this glowing truth of your Love as it dances between you, you will speed up the world and reveal its truth. It will also spread easily to all other humans because, by your light, they will be able to see. So as Jesus brought forth an awareness of your nature with which to light the world, you will now take that light within you and use it to see your SoulMate. Jesus regained the truth of his SoulMate, and he used that light to illuminate the world. Now it is time that each of you experiences this. If his experience was enough to revolutionize human thinking (which it was), *just think what it will mean as millions of SoulMates give forth their light – the light that is the result of the movement of their Love!*

So by itself, with no conscious action on your parts, just the experience of your reunion with your SoulMates can completely and totally change the world. Now add to this your conscious co-creation. Then you will see that our beloved humanity can easily be awakened and this precious and beautiful Earth returned to its true reality of rich, verdant life and beauty. You will recognize the grace of the SoulMate awakening coming now, just in time. You will see that the fact that the SoulMate heart, the awakened and reunified human being, can do nothing else but turn to the tender upliftment of humankind and planet.

And just to give you this last important piece to keep you expanding, I ask you to remember that since you, humanity, are the embodiment of all Love in form, this beautiful planet is a part of you. As you surrender to the awakening of your reunion, as you allow the phoenix of the SoulMate union to rise from the ashes of the ego relationship, the Earth and all life within and upon it will rise with you. Perfectly. Automatically. Love is once again illuminated by the light of Love's movement, which is the cause and the result of the reunion of SoulMates.

Oh, do not worry if this is difficult to comprehend. It will become clear to you. It will become clear as you invite My presence to illuminate you. For as it moves more and more fully into your life, light will shine into you and it will illuminate everything.

41

I ask you now, this very moment, to invite Me. Invite Me into you, into your life, into your world. And know as you do this that absolutely everything in your life will be illuminated in My presence. All things within you that may be blocking your awakening, the recognition of your SoulMate, or the perfect return to your embodiment of Love will be revealed. Effortlessly. Gently. Remember this, for I Am Love. I will never hurt you in the name of Love. *So if you find yourself suffering through the process of growing, you can be assured that your ego has gotten between us.*

Elevation. Elevation is the process by which the truth of Love is understood. It is the speeding up of vibration until your consciousness is vibrating fast enough to mesh with the truth of Love. Life on the physical plane, of course, is vibrating very slowly. Slowly enough that things appear and are experienced as solid. This is very slow. *So to embrace the truth of Love, to understand it, you must vibrate fast enough to connect with it.* You could picture this as gears. The tools that you use to accomplish elevation are the opposite of a clutch. Rather than slowing down a wheel that it may mesh, you must speed up so your consciousness will mesh with the faster moving truth. All of your prayers, affirmations and meditations are for this purpose, and they are very important. However, *the fastest way to elevate the speed or the rate of vibration of your consciousness is the reunion with your SoulMate.* For then, dear ones, you are rejoined as the heart of Love. Immediately. This happens the moment you surrender your heart into the SoulMate union.

This union is the "elevator." It will take you up immediately to the vibrational level of truth, of real Love. It is the entryway to the Christ Consciousness for humanity. The Christ is, as I have continually told you, the manifestation of My Love. Thus you can now see how the "Second Coming of Christ," the raising up meant for this time of humanity, is to be claimed, experienced through the reunion of SoulMates.

There are many others who have stated that the coming together of SoulMates would herald the Golden Age. This is true. It is far truer than you can yet imagine.

I have painted the biggest picture — the vast stage of the cosmos and the movement of Love within it that is your destiny. I also must remind you that I am fully present in all things in this glorious Creation that is My being. Thus, My beloved ones, I can be as vast as the great All. I can expand you and expand you until you can touch the very edges of Creation itself. And I can be intimate. Oh, so deeply present in your life that I speak with absolute clarity within you. Of course this is true because I am everything, including your loving parent, your most tender support, and your greatest encouragement. Thus I am both the teacher and the one who is taught. *You can bring anything to Me to place in the light of My loving presence and I will reveal its truth.*

Because you are co-creators, together with each other you are the plus and minus moving upon the substance of My being. As well as lifting your consciousness to the apex – the moment of Creation – you can also allow the pure light to pour down through your being to illuminate everything encountered. This is the experience (the commitment) of those of you who have offered to uplift this pseudo reality — to bring the knowledge of your real essence back into full view. The light is poured through these SoulMates to bless and illuminate and to transform the lower vibrations that are creating this false reality. At this moment there is great need for this. However, this could change very quickly as people are reconnected to their truth and as SoulMates use the commitment of their unified heart to simply melt away the illusion.

Thus, while I will call you all to this service of transformation and though it may be temporarily intense and very necessary, I ask that within it you continually hold the vision of the truth of Love and of the power of the forces of Creation brought into this dimension by the reunified SoulMates. This way you will always be grounded (or uplifted, actually) in the truth of Love. There is nothing more important.

I make one more promise to you, My beloved, precious humanity. If you will do the work of getting past the ego and into the heart, I will always demonstrate the truth and the power of Love. I will always demonstrate the reality of SoulMates. With each demonstration you will become more and more connected with the truth of your Love, the reality of your SoulMate, and the glory of knowing that you are the embodiment of the relationship of the movement of Love that is the creative force.

Together with your SoulMate, you are the heart of another universe. Come through this doorway now, reach out, open your heart, and you will know what it means to be My heart.

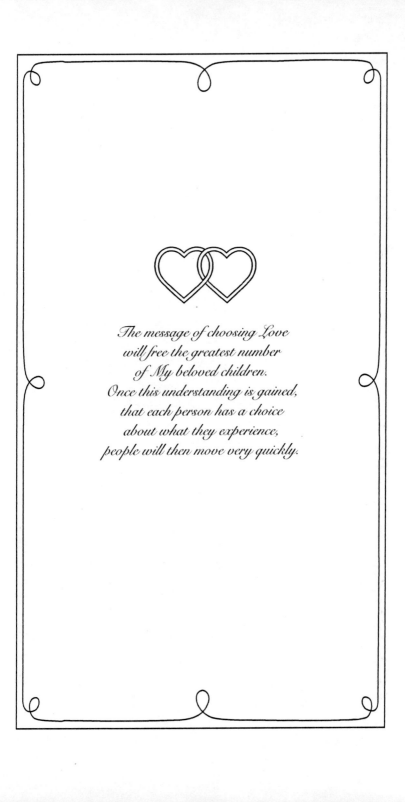

The message of choosing Love
will free the greatest number
of My beloved children.
Once this understanding is gained,
that each person has a choice
about what they experience,
people will then move very quickly.

The Womb of Creation

I am here with you. It is good for you to sit, tuned to Me, open, receptive and waiting to receive. This is different from praying. Prayer is outward moving energy. It is the use of your Will as well as your Love. Meditation – ah! Meditation is tapping into the great creative moment, the stillness before life is born. Meditation is an important key to the work of co-creation, for first you must receive. You must create the empty Womb of Creation between you and your SoulMate, holding it in the silence for My blessing, and for the receptivity needed to draw forward the elements of life for you to direct with your consciousness.

When you feel that you can't meditate, that your mind will not be stilled, or when others say this to you, here is what I suggest. Become the feminine, the receiver of life. Assume the position of waiting to be impregnated with the new — new light, new energy, the ingredients for the quickening, the birth of new life. Focus your mind if you cannot still it, and you will also create the room needed for the spirit to penetrate you.

You have heard for many years that every being is androgynous, containing both male and female. First, I will say that most of the time this reasoning is used as an excuse for not opening to the SoulMate, for not believing that your counterpart could manifest outside of you. So, people have focused on making this an inner event. In truth, dear ones, it is not.

Now this is going to shatter some very cherished illusions, but they must be shattered. It is time to realize this.

Each of you is a ray of God. Ultimately, each of you is either the male or the female energy. There are definite charges, definite energy. Just as there are the seven rays of color, so there are the positive charge (masculine) and negative charge (feminine) rays as they pour forth from Me. These are the creative power. It is the interaction of the positive and the negative charges that is the spark of Creation. And while the expressions of your many selves experiencing the learning through many worlds (many incarnations) can wear both male and female bodies, ultimately you are only one. At the level of Creation, at the level of SoulMates, your opposite is outside of you, not inside.

Thus I say to all of you, please raise your vision. As you do, you will see your beautiful glorious SoulMate. Because of your polarities, your SoulMate creates a life force between you, a life force that is the energy of Creation. Together you do learn how to use both the positive and the negative energy. You learn how to penetrate with your Will, how to charge forth in the way of male energy, and you learn how to open up, to nourish life, to welcome the penetration, how to tenderly support the growth of the new in the way of the feminine energy. But learning how to *use* these energies, dear ones, is different from *being* these energies.

Before you are awake, it is easy to identify with the outer sheath, the body with which you clothe yourself. Thus you believe that you are male energy because you wear a male body, female energy because you wear a female body. But deep within there is a greater truth. This is the truth of your being, who you are in the moment of your creation as you moved forth into existence in My heart. In that truth, you are one half of a cell, the other half being your SoulMate. *From the moment of your conception as a point of My Love, you are one energy, female or male.*

As you choose your SoulMate and allow the rest of you to manifest, you will see clearly who you are at Creation level. If you don't already know, you probably sense or strongly suspect the truth of your charge, masculine or feminine. Now, you must learn to use both the positive and negative energies, and it can work for you at this level, and work well, to see these energies as part of your being. But as you choose to move to the next level, to welcome your SoulMate into your life, it is important to release this helpful tool and examine who you truly are.

For once you know if you are the plus or the minus, the positive or the negative, the masculine or the feminine, then you know how the divine energy comes into Creation through you. It is then that you know just how the Love that I pour forth through each cell of My heart (each SoulMate couple) is to manifest through you. Once you know this, then you will know how to wield that energy.

You will use this energy to bless and heal the world because when you accept it fully, and only when you do, you will be polarized enough to create the spark of life between you and your SoulMate, and only when you can create the spark of life can you become co-creators.

So the myth of androgyny must now be released. The glorious acceptance of your divine nature, of which half of the ray of Love you embody, now becomes critical for you and for the world. Once you allow yourselves to fully embody what you are, masculine or feminine, you will be able to align yourself with the Divine Mother or Divine Father light. It is only through the interaction of these two lights that Creation appears.

If you have only one, say only the divine positive, shining forth from the point of light that is the beginning of

Creation, there is nothing that can be seen. Even if things are there, they are invisible! It requires the contrasting light to bring them into view. This is not dark and light – please do not make that mistake. No, these lights are exactly this, the opposite ends of the spectrum, between which All That Is (which is all of Me) can be seen.

Dear ones, this may not mean much to you now, but very quickly it will. To move your world from invisible to visible (to the rest of the cosmos) it will require the awakened masculine and feminine energies (in other words, the SoulMates). As some of you have glimpsed, Sacred Geometry verifies this also – that Creation comes forth as the joining of the male and the female. Always that is how it is. The idea of both energies being present in one being is only of assistance only at a certain stage of development. Here, particularly in the current ego culture (listen carefully), the topic of having it all within has been co-opted by the ego to discourage you from pursuing true Love. (By now you realize that true Love is the true end of the ego's existence!)

Of course, I place these things before you with My request to say "yes" to your SoulMate. This I must do, for it is a necessity. But I also want you to realize, those of you who already accept this, that this knowledge of energies is integral to learning how to create.

So now, you have the awareness that your SoulMate is part of you, as you are part of him/her. The illusion cannot change this. Your acceptance of this truth will clear the path for this awakening for you. Whether or not your SoulMate has manifested before you, you can begin to work with the laws and the path of co-creation. As you do, your sureness will allow your SoulMate to fully embody with you.

As you know, there are endless possibilities to the experience of Love, to the awakening of the SoulMate relationship, and to your blossoming into co-creatorship. But I tell you that truth is truth, and you can enter into relationship with truth at every point on the continuum of consciousness as long as there is awareness of Me and acceptance of Love. I ask all of you to take in this statement, to deeply embrace it and make it a part of you. For once you understand this one thing, you will have moved beyond judgment. Dearest ones, life is a hologram, meaning that I am fully present in every part.

Knowing this, I ask you to realize that the gift of awareness belongs to everyone. I say this to you passionately, and with urgency. It does not belong only to those with a "high consciousness." Yes, a higher vibration allows for an experience of truth more clearly (pay attention), but that does not mean it is any more true. It is so very important that all of you grasp this.

A hologram means that the whole is present in all of the parts. Thus, someone who can barely make out the truth is nonetheless seeing that truth if they have decided to look for it in Love. It is still Me, even if seen "through a glass darkly." *Knowing this, I ask that you who are more awake do everything you possibly can to provide access to truth to those who are less awake, for if they can touch it at all, purely, they are actually touching it all.*

I will now give you simple ways to access the truth of SoulMates, simple ways to experience and identify the truth of Love, as well as ways more complex and esoteric. I ask you to remember to make no judgments that one is better than the other.

Your SoulMate is part of you whether or not you can see him/her. So here is a first glimpse at co-creation, simply and lovingly placed before you, that all of you may begin to understand your truth — that you are the cells of My Heart.

Thus as I create, so do you, and now you can begin to do so consciously. It takes the male and female energy, on every level of Creation (not just here) to do this. I speak here of energies, not the bodies containing the energy.

Step One: Discern if, at the level of your being, you are female or male energy.

Step Two: Fully accept and embody this energy, more and more and more, until you can sense the connection of this energy in you, going all the way up to original Creation, the "First Split Ray." Allow yourself to become a vehicle for the Divine Mother or the Divine Father light.

Step Three: Get together with your SoulMate on whatever level you can make contact. This contact can be an intuitive sense. It can even be just an affirmation of your surety that your SoulMate is with you.

Step Four: Join your hearts (the critical step! Do not ever leave it out or you may end up creating "anti-Love" energy.)

Step Five: Connect your chakras.

Step Six: See that together your chakras and energies uniting create a Double Helix of energy movement.

Step Seven: Create a Womb of Creation between your two hearts. Your Double Helix intersects there. Your energy bodies are joined into One there.

Step Eight: Meditate together. Allow full receptivity to make your Womb of Creation fertile and ready to receive life. Join with Divine Mother.

Step Nine: Plant the seed. Speak aloud what you are planting. Connect with the Divine Father, the penetrating light, knowing it is this light that has the power of planting the seed.

Step Ten: Feed or fertilize your creation (your "pregnancy"). Do this by each of you fully allowing your femaleness or maleness to become an open channel for the Divine Female or Divine Male. Be sure that the energy pouring from you into your Womb of Creation is coming from Source, from the highest level of female or male, from the point where these energies move forth from Me into Creation. This step is as important as joining your hearts.

Step Eleven: Bring your creation to the physical plane. Do this by taking time to visualize (and speak if you like, which will reinforce it) your creation as clearly as possible as it will appear in the world. Feel it. Experience it. If you have difficulty doing this, describe verbally exactly what it will feel like, look like, how you will experience it. This step brings the energy down the vibrational scale and anchors it here. This is what most people know of as manifestation or co-creation. After you have done this,

Step Twelve: Speak the words of Power. Together (very important) visualize your throat chakras joined together, as part of that Double Helix that is your SoulMate energy. Then together say, "It is created. It is now done." (Be sure to say "now" unless you specifically want it to wait to manifest. Though it can be tricky at this level of information, you can determine when on the time line you want something to appear.) You can add any other powerful and definitive words of affirmation.

This, dear ones, is the creative power of SoulMates. Whenever someone is working on manifestation on their own, it draws their SoulMate to them – always. Thus, if your SoulMate is not yet in view, one of the best ways to begin the relationship, to start the process of their manifestation, is to begin to co-create.

I give you here a very great gift. Please do not take this lightly. Approach this, and everything to do with your SoulMate with the greatest reverence and gratitude. I tell you, it is the greatest gift that I could give you, to create you thus. You will always have what I lacked – a consciousness before you who can reflect to you your truth, who can show yourself to you, the embodiment of the greatest truth of all, the truth of Love.

This is the reason I created you, out of My longing for that very same reflective consciousness. When you have grown, this is what you will be to Me — collectively, as the one being that is humanity, and individually as the cells of My heart. It is your journey into experience, as you know, that always has been the way by which I also experience every possibility of Myself. Through you I know about myself. Through you I have even examined the thought of a world without Love. This is the darkness that you have endured. And through you I have grown and continue to grow, to expand My Creation and My Creatorship, a blessing beyond your capability to understand at this moment. Yet, of course, in truth you understand perfectly. You have never left My heart. But you have **dreamed** that you have, and through those dreams I have grown My own heart.

I pour My blessings on you, and I urgently nudge you while I whisper, "Awake!" for you are becoming a new being as your SoulMate DNA comes together as ever more glorious Love. I am with you, especially as you seek to understand.

Remember that you already know, and enjoy the beautiful experience of remembering.

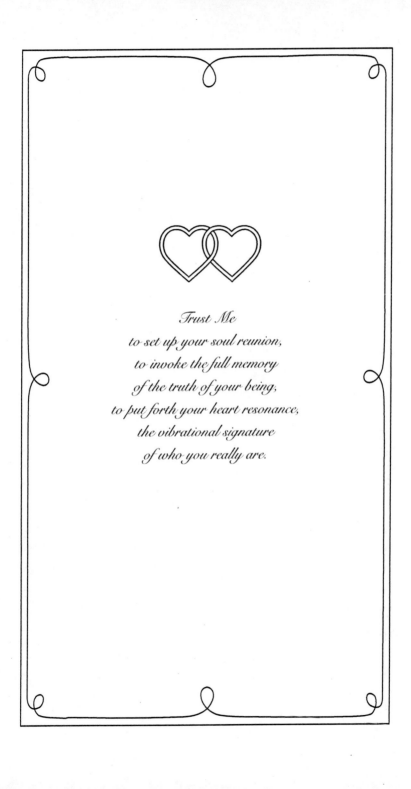

Trust Me
to set up your soul reunion,
to invoke the full memory
of the truth of your being,
to put forth your heart resonance,
the vibrational signature
of who you really are.

Divine Feminine and Divine Masculine, Believing That Love is Worth Everything

The Divine Feminine holds the Love. The Divine Feminine supports every part of Creation as it is meant to be. Then, when you add the counterpart, the Divine Masculine, then you have movement!

When creation began within Me, first it was an idea. It rose within Me. It was an idea to create life, to manifest Love perfectly. This thought was the first self-awareness of the Divine Feminine. The first part was the rising up within Me of all the images of perfection. I saw how it would be if all the elements within Me came forth. These images were held in perfect surrender to the magnificence of the whole image.

The second part was the movement. The masculine energy came streaking in and moved the sacred images, the true presence, into form. Then the perfect images had life, for the masculine energy penetrated. In that penetration, it sparked! That spark began the process that built energy until new life emerged.

This process is true on all levels. Whether it is an entire creation or whether it is a physical sperm entering a physical egg, creating new life. First, I held in Love within Me an idea, all parts suspending themselves in the sea of Love that is My consciousness. This was phase one of the "First Split," the plus, the womb, the circle, the held breath that contains all things. Then, I willed it to be SO! Movement. My energy rose up and up in the desire to express all that was within Me. The second phase of the "First Split" occurred. From the One there came Two, the positive and the negative. There came the circle, the womb, and the line, the arrow, the Will which gives direction, stirring the ethers of the womb and bringing forth life. New life.

All creation that is alive, moving, growing, expanding, is alive as a result of these two energies. Thus, we come to the awakening of humankind and the crucial nature of the SoulMate couples.

Dear ones, although Creation is ever-evolving through the interaction of these energies, this is a time when their use is critical. For to understand what must be brought forth in Love, the idea must be held perfectly in the greatest, most tender devotion by the Divine Feminine. Then it must be sparked into life by the Divine Masculine.

This is why you are now on Earth. You cannot look at the outer shell, or the human vehicle to understand who and what you are. This I promise you. As you accept the capacity you have and the service you have come to do, you will discover direct acknowledgment of the truth of your being continually. All you have to do is open to it. You will find the beings that serve humanity, be they Masters or angels, greeting you as equals. You will find all of Nature fully acknowledging you. If you open honestly, with true humility (not the false humility of ego), you will find the verification all around you.

Now as you understand what it means to embody this energy, the Divine Feminine and the Divine Masculine, at the highest level you can possibly reach, you will understand easily just what you are holding in your consciousness for creation.

In other words, you will be able to take in from all of life the perfection of the expression of each and every being. Then, you will open yourself to Me completely and thus you will know the perfection of humanity. Now you are the womb. The circle containing the new creation. Held within you is the blueprint of the New World.

Then you will turn and deliver yourself, in complete trust, to your SoulMate for quickening. The template of Creation held within you will be brought to life by the one who holds the masculine energy, the movement, the penetration, the spark. The New World, the perfected humanity, the perfect expression of every part of this creation will come to life!

At every step of the way, as consciousness is expanded, the principle of creation is the same. So, as SoulMate couples are drawn back together, with any conscious awareness at all, they will greatly contribute to the shift, or the awakening. First, I ask you to simply accept this truth of your beings – that you are the perfect expression of the Divine Feminine or the Divine Masculine. Then raise your consciousness, if you can, until you receive confirmation from life, Nature, the Ascended Masters. Don't make this difficult. Don't make it great big. Just fit yourself into it, until you know it is right for you. Then begin to co-create. This will bring much learning to you.

Just realize that you, the SoulMate couples, have an important part of the greatest Love story ever told. Also know that, whether they know it consciously or not, all of humankind has been searching for this story – not only for all of this life, but for all of their lives since "The Fall." Before "The Fall" you were with your SoulMates, living in the full consciousness of Love. The biblical story of Adam and Eve is actually a very accurate rendering, using symbology, of the loss of the awareness of your SoulMate.

I want you to go in and release that dream. Bring it back out into the light. Say to everyone, "This is the most important dream you can have. Do not give up! Do not back down! *Do not believe that Love isn't worth everything – worth fighting for."*

I am with you. We are ready to make our precious humanity's dreams come true.

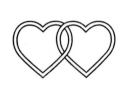

So, by itself,
with no conscious action on your parts,
just the experience of your reunion
with your SoulMates
can completely and totally change the world.
Now add to this your conscious co-creation.
Then you will see that
our beloved humanity can easily be awakened
and this precious and beautiful Earth returned
to its true reality of rich, verdant life and beauty.

Divine Feminine
and Divine Masculine Together
Create a Wholeness of Christ

Beloveds, please listen. It is the stretching forth of Divine Love Feminine that will be the blanketing Love, the tender hand that will reach out to the hearts of My children. The truth is that humanity is hungry for the balancing feminine energy, especially in the industrialized nations, for *this feminine energy is the energy of unity. It is the force of Love that draws people together as family, be this individual family or the family of humankind.* The Divine Love Feminine is the force of Love that is embodied in Nature, in the Earth, which again people desperately need.

As you fully allow this Divine Feminine energy to bless and awaken you, the connection that you have to all of life will also become fully alive. Your days will become a true celebration, and a joyous exchange. For especially here, in the Western world, people have been flooded with judgment in the name of spirituality. In the name of Christianity, the majority of people have been threatened with terrible things if a judgment is passed and they are found unworthy. Since the energy of the Divine Feminine is so very loving and so obviously without any judgment, many people will be drawn to it that have not been able to continue to function in the distortion of Christ's message.

Most importantly, it is true that now *the Divine Feminine must come in to correct the imbalance of the last 2000 years.* Everything in this Western culture is moving around a distorted Divine Male energy. There is a great need for people to re-absorb the Divine Feminine and to find a place in their lives for it. This you will all help anchor here. The true Divine Feminine is vast – expansive beyond measure – while filled with such complete and unconditional Love that its warmth and tenderness completely wraps every being. It is Love as it moves forth in blessing. It is larger than what is perceived by the pagan community. Yet those who worship there are definitely responding first to the call of the Divine Feminine. Through the Divine Feminine, I will give My greatest tenderness, My completely powerful encircling of every human being, the complete and total unconditional Love and acceptance that I hold for My beloved humanity.

Dear ones, as long as there is judgment of any kind there cannot be real Love. I want My beloveds to know that truth of My Love for them — that it is totally complete. Absolutely unconditional. I am filled with awe at your beauty, each and every one of you. Only when a person can allow this kind of Love will he or she be able to fully experience My Love for them.

The coming of the Christ in this age is the perfect embodiment of the Divine Masculine and the Divine Feminine into the wholeness of Christ. It is to be a Love that contains the perfectly balanced masculine and feminine energies at the Christ level. People have sensed this, or received this information, but have long interpreted it as becoming androgynous. You will find this theory put forth regularly by those who are carrying great quantities of light, those who are truly sensing the advent of these balancing energies. But without the awareness of the truth of SoulMates, they have no way to explain it but to say it must be within one person.

In truth, it is not possible for both forces to be fully present in one person. It is not possible because, as you know, you each have a Divine Nature. You have either a positive or a negative charge to your being, as half of a whole cell in My heart.

I think this is a good time to mention again what we have touched on before. *These charges do not necessarily correspond to current physical bodies.* As you know, beings change gender continually as they come to learn specific things. Normally those who are spiritually evolved will wear a body consistent with their divine charge. Thus a person who has had a last few lives of awakening will most likely have all of them in their natural or divine gender. But for a number of reasons, this may not always be the case, the biggest of these being the urgent need to move beyond judgment. *Those who have incarnated in same sex bodies will have in their lives people who will be opened by the experience of exposure to the couple.*

There are also other reasons for SoulMates to incarnate as same sex couples. So it is important to be clear in presenting the SoulMate information that we are not necessarily speaking of heterosexual couples. You have long pondered why same sex couples almost always have a very masculine person and a feminine person. This is why. A couple will always be a plus and a minus, a positive and a negative energy, a masculine and a feminine energy. Now *that* is a cosmic law. It is not because of any judgment. *It is simply about magnetism and the facts of creation. Plus and minus attract. Two of the same charge repel – just as you find with magnets.* If reincarnation had been left in the Bible, the correct interpretation of this cosmic fact would be possible for everyone studying the Bible. They could then understand that it is not about the body people are wearing in each lifetime, but about the charge of their spirit.

Remember how I said that a relatively small number of conscious SoulMate couples can affect a big change? It is because you are the embodiment of the energy of Creation.

Completely. Once understood, you will have the full force of these "First Split," or first movement energies to direct.

Dear ones, seek continually to hold the perfect Love of these divine energies, that they can spark recognition in all human hearts. If not recognition of SoulMates, then of the truth of Love. If not recognition of the truth of Love, then the value of giving. If not the value of giving, the precious enfoldment by My Love of the human family. In other words, while awakening those who can hear the trumpet call of the New World, we must reach every heart in some way. In this time, Love will multiply exponentially every day, and we must accomplish those points of entry to every being.

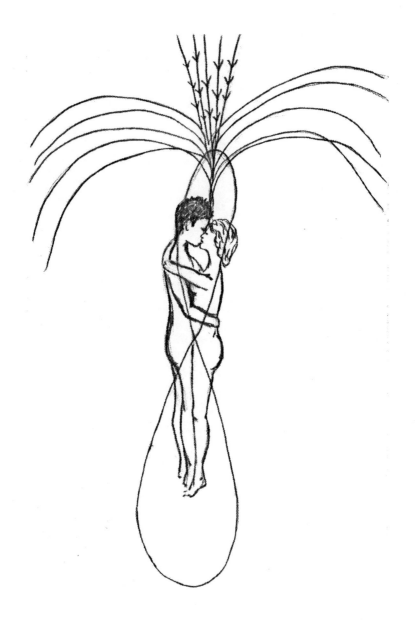

Under the Wings of Your Love

Uniting with Your SoulMate
A Love Beyond Eternal

My beloved ones who are My blessed heart and whose eyes are now lifting to the vision of your possibilities, I have come to stretch you again. I have come to point your hearts at a greater Love and to seal them in the glorious truth of your SoulMates. Oh, dear ones, there is so much Love waiting to pour through you! There is so much Love waiting to be recognized – recognized as your own — seen in your SoulMate's eyes.

There is indeed a world to save. But even greater than this, there is an awakening in your hearts of the certainty of Love – that Love is the basis of every single atom, the truth of your deepest nature. There must now develop a similar surety – now that you are uniting with your SoulMate at the level of Creation, that you together will become a force of Love, ready to bring forth your own creation in Me.

Now I must answer questions that have arisen and will continue to arise as the words of the promise of your SoulMate penetrates your consciousness. First, though, I must tell you that whatever you don't understand I ask that you hold it in your heart, bathe it in your Love and wait. In its time it will reveal to you every answer on every level of Creation.

Now you are often looking at your SoulMate as you would look at a physical plane mate. But I must tell you that this union is far bigger than anything you could ever encounter here. I encourage you to dream, dream of everything that represents to you the greatest Love you can possibly imagine. Then I promise you, it is more, more than all you have ever imagined, more than the most cherished, secret dreams of Love. It is more than any fairy tale, better than any possible imagination. *Not only is your SoulMate your equivalent in every way, but your Love is beyond eternal.*

People have asked questions about a person that they were receiving as their SoulMate, but who was married to another person, or showed no interest, or was not available to them for some reason. I will answer this question and in the process I will attempt to get through to you an inkling of the great truth of your SoulMate.

First let me speak on the most obvious level - that of the person on the physical plane. *I will tell you unequivocally that if a person is for any reason not available, that person is not your expression of your SoulMate. You can also be absolutely sure that there is a message in the appearance in your life of one who carries your SoulMate's energy, but who is unavailable for whatever reason.*

Dear ones, this is a clear message that your SoulMate is near, for you are being drawn to his energy, but *there is something in you that is keeping him away.* There is a reason you have made him appear close, but really far away – tantalizing you with the great recognition, yes, but far enough away for "safety." *Most of the time the reason for this is your fear.* You want your Love but you are at the same time afraid. You are still carrying the memories of previous pain and you're not yet willing to let it go. For whatever reason, you are not allowing your SoulMate to actually come to you.

Opening to your SoulMate will never, and I repeat, NEVER, break up another relationship. That is not how Love works. That is a very, very limited vision of Love to think there is not enough to go around so you must take something from another. Please do not ever use ego games to justify any action that is out of integrity with life, with Love, for in doing so, you would cut off your growth right there, at the ego level. *A relationship begun with pain to another, or with someone who is not finished where they are, cannot ever be the basis for true SoulMate union or Sacred Sexuality.* You can be assured, dear ones, that if someone is still in a relationship, regardless of the ego's tales of woe, that person is not complete. They are not finished. They are not awake. If they were awake and ready to be the vehicle of your SoulMate union, they would be free and ready.

Now here is where I must ask you to stretch, for, dearest ones, it is very important. If you are ready to embrace such a great truth as your SoulMate, you must also embrace the great truth of your being. You must begin to open yourself to the real nature of Love, and the completely transcendent nature of your very being. Only thus can you begin to see large enough to be worthy of your SoulMate Love and to be able to use it to create. You must have a big enough vision to be able to use such a glorious relationship for the healing and awakening of the world.

As you have learned, you only have one SoulMate. This SoulMate is the other half of your great and glorious eternal being. This SoulMate is the other half, with you, of the cell of My heart. This being is that cell born into manifestation at the moment of Creation, for in that moment I became manifested. I became the expanding Creation, of which you are the heart. The essence of that moment, when thought moved upon the deep ocean of My being, was the creation of Divine Masculine and Divine Feminine.

Until that moment I was still consciousness. A pool of Love. But there rose in Me the great desire to give forth that Love. This desire grew within Me until it burst forth and, crackling with the energy of My longing, it became two things instead of one. It became the giver and the one who receives. Out of this moment and this action upon the deep, the action of Will, of thought, upon the ocean of My Love, My Love brought forth All That Is. All That Is in relationship. *All That Is in relationship is forever comprised of the energies of the "First Split," where that which receives became the Divine Feminine and that which gives, the Divine Masculine. Thus everything in Creation is now and forever the relationship of these two energies, including the nature of the cells of My heart.*

That, dear ones, was the creation of SoulMates. That moment. Those two energies that have now been manifested through every level. It is always the same, always the one relationship – two halves of one cell of My heart equals SoulMates. This is the SoulMate I am talking about. This is the being I ask you to call forth into your life. Not just your life partner. Not just your equivalent. Not just someone who will help you grow or teach you things. No! *I want you to ask for your true and glorious SoulMate, also referred to as your Twin Flame.*

Now you have all heard about various divisions, levels of SoulMates, and you have even been told that these were all different beings. They are not. You have one SoulMate. Always. Forever. However, that SoulMate has had many manifestations.

Here is where I must stretch you. I ask you to open and to accept this on faith until your own faculties can, and will, prove it to you. I ask you to accept no other than your true SoulMate. But before you begin to lament that this person is not in your life or out of your reach, or even married to someone else, let Me explain. Please take this in the best you can.

You are each a cell in the heart of God. I ask you now to do your very best to imagine what this means. Stretch! Think! Well, if God is Creator of All That Is, then within God is everything that exists. This includes millions of galaxies and worlds within worlds and beings unlimited in their vastness and scope. Now if this is the truth of Me, your beloved Creator, then how big *is* My heart? The answer – huge beyond your imagining! This is you and your SoulMate! You are great and glorious and vast beyond your imagining! And just as in Me I created all through the relationship of the masculine and feminine, just so are you and your SoulMate also able to create. Not little things, dear ones. Worlds. Galaxies. Civilizations of life forms formed from your union.

Knowing this, that the truth of you and your SoulMate is huge, I ask you to see your life now from that perspective. *You, in your manifestation here, are a tiny little splinter of the vast being that you are.* You are manifested here, though, which is a very big thing. It means you are in the process of awakening to your presence in My heart.

Now I have explained to you before about the problem that we had in the beginning. It was this. You loved Me so much (and I, you) that you could not stay away from Me. You could not become individualized because you would blissfully sink back into the Love that we are.

Knowing it was our goal to relate (the whole reason for Creation), you, the great beings who are My heart, chose to move away from Me, to individuate, so you could become your own identity. So (pay attention), you turned and dove outward into Creation, moving down into density to gain distance from Me. It was the only way we could do it. As you dove, you looked out at all of these levels you went through on your outward journey. Every time you looked, a piece of your attention/consciousness took up residence at that level in order to explore it. These are what we call your incarnations, or personalities.

This Earth level was the end of the dive, if you want to look at it this way. So on all these various levels of experience, there are pieces of your consciousness all existing at once, and all in contact with the higher self. However, things became very dense here at this last level of your manifested lives, and you lost contact with all of the other pieces of consciousness. It can be likened to being on a Star Trek away mission. You are down here on the planet. You've lost communication with the ship. You think you are alone and you are caught in a "temporal anomaly," so it seems you have been here forever. All the while, the crew is aware of everything you do and is desperately trying to get a message through with instructions on how to get back to the ship.

Now your SoulMate is the great, vast being who is huge, as are you. While both of you have had your attention placed outward on these personalities through your many incarnations to build your separate identities, you are still who you are. Your SoulMate is still vast and powerful and so are you. It is this energy, this real fullness of your SoulMate you are now returning to. For the personalities have served their purpose. They have created many experiences and strong and individualized beings of the two of you. Now it is time for the two great energies that you are to reunite.

Dear ones, there is no way to fully explain to you the truth of this vastness of your being. Suffice it so say that the two of you, Twin Rays, great SoulMates of the "First Split" of My being, will now send forth the truth of your beings. This truth will pour through every one of your many personalities or incarnations and all of them will recognize the truth of who they really are and call forth the connection with the true, vast, great and powerful fullness of their true being.

In other words, every personality being expressed by your great self will now be lifted into the truth. As the great being pours through you more and more and more, the personalities you were will be lifted up vibrationally and expanded until they become a part of the Great SoulMate Union.

This is why I have said to you that your SoulMate will manifest through the person you are with. For *I guarantee that in every incarnation, every person you have ever been with is a piece of your SoulMate. Every one. And in every incarnation your SoulMate has been reflecting to you your state of consciousness.* It is always your SoulMate, wearing different personalities to mirror to you the state of your Love. It is only because you are way down in this density that you can believe that it is different people. Once you really understand the truth, you will realize that such a thought is absurd.

If you are cells of My heart which contain only one positive and one negative charge, then everyone you relate to can only be the other half of that cell of My heart. Once you truly understand the truth of your SoulMate, you will see it perfectly. If your SoulMate is ever and always with you, yet you must learn how to be individualized through the illusion and then return to Love, the only way it could be done is for each of you to wear many personalities, each helping the other to grow into full consciousness of Love as individualized cells of My heart.

Many of you reading this are going to recognize it. "Oh, yes! Of course!," your heart will say. Many of you have had the experience of meeting someone and knowing his/her spirit. And feeling this, you could have sworn, "this was it" – only to find that your personalities could not get along at all, that your egos had a heyday. This is because you did know them. Their *essence* was your SoulMate, but you were not

75

open enough to Love to draw in the truth of your SoulMate. For as you now see, *it is only as you become Love that Love will become what you see and what you live.*

So if you meet someone and you know that person is your SoulMate, she may be. But, if the person does not reflect Love back to you, I can promise you that it is a message for you to see why you are holding Love at bay. Why you are protecting yourself, and so forth. I also can promise you that in such a case you are very close to ready, because you have actually drawn yourself right to one of your SoulMate's personalities. This should be cause for celebration. It should also be cause for deep, deep self-examination and loving, but ruthless self-honesty. Then, as soon as you have worked through what was blocking you, someone will appear through whom your SoulMate can truly manifest.

As you awaken, you open your beings. Your SoulMate manifests with you, still as a personality. As you expand, more and more of the light that is your great SoulMate self pours into the two of you. You become less and less defined on this physical plane as your beings become more and more comprised of the great Love that you are. You also become ever more conscious of who you really are and how you really relate as great SoulMates. Eventually your physical selves are "spiritualized," actually becoming the substance of your true SoulMate selves, which is, in truth, the very substance of My heart. At this point, you are totally transformed and the matter that you were wearing as bodies, living in as personalities and touching with your consciousness, is also transformed into that same substance of the Love of My heart.

I realize this is a lot to take in for some of you. For others it will seem as if you always knew. But whether or not you can fully grasp the implications, I ask you to completely trust the truth of Love. That truth is your SoulMate, one being forever, wearing many personalities. Together, you are a cell in My very heart. I ask you to know that the purity of Love in your heart and your call for your SoulMate pours the golden light of your highest self down into your life, and the more you can accept it as your truth the more you will see it in your world. Your SoulMate will manifest ever more clearly as you are clear and able to see Love. Your SoulMate has manifested that personality you see before you. Absolutely. In reflection of your own Love.

Do not allow your ego to convince you differently or you will lose precious time. Instead, look up. Acknowledge the highest truth of your SoulMate relationship as My heart. Hold yourself in perfect Love so you can see through the illusion of what you think is in front of you and you will find the truth of SoulMate Love, drawn perfectly into your life by the clarity of your consciousness and by the remembrance of who you are.

I ask you now to live your highest vision. The highest integrity. The most reverence for Love. The full ecstatic experience of giving that will align you with My being. Then, when you have carefully ascertained what is the very highest you can reach, reach higher. Trust your SoulMate's existence and manifestation ever more fully in your life, completely. Live by this trust without question. Look for the truth of both of you in your partner's eyes. And know, dear ones, that *you do not need to go anywhere to find your SoulMate. You have never been apart.* If you are with someone, begin right now to see the truth. Begin to love so purely that the highest level of your being can be delivered to both of you. Live expectantly and greet every increase in Love and energy with celebration and joy. Then turn together and begin generating Love for the world that the clouds of illusion for everyone will be melted away in the sunshine of your Love.

Catch hold of this vision, dear ones, and live it every day. You will quickly find that you have never imagined even a fraction of the joy and the out-pouring of Love that is the union with your SoulMate. *Let Me tell you that every couple in the world today should be experiencing this amazing awakening to Love.* Anyone who complains of being bored or unfulfilled is not listening to his/her heart.

The greatest key for the reclamation of the SoulMate Love is giving. This you can do no matter what the illusion has placed before you. If you can't see this possibility in your partner, start speaking to his spirit, for I promise that your spirits are SoulMates, are glory and communion of Love. As you open your heart, you will see your SoulMate. This I promise you.

So all who are looking, must look within themselves, that they will be clear enough to receive the Love being sent from the highest level of their beings, the SoulMate as Divine Masculine or Divine Feminine. If you can "unfreeze" yourself, your SoulMate will follow. And should you find yourself with a seemingly recalcitrant personality, I ask you to not be fooled by appearances. Know that Love will find a way. *Your SoulMate's truth will be seen by you to the degree that you are able to see it in yourself, to give it to your partner, and to see it as their highest truth.* Remember, Love is expansion. Giving is Love's truth. Judgment is the annihilator of Love's precious growth.

I am with you, beloveds, teaching you your greatest truth.

I ask you to
***Trust Love**.*
Trust Love to evolve your relationship.
Trust Love to refine your vibrations,
to accelerate your consciousness
and to evolve your Love Making.
Trust Love with all your being,
with all of your
heart and soul and dedication,
and Love will open like a rose
within the two of you together,
revealing the trust
of all Creation.

Across the Divide,
SoulMates Recreate the World

Before "The Fall," human couples knew. They knew what they embodied. They knew pure Love, yes. But they knew pure Love exactly as it is at the "First Split." They knew what it meant to be the embodiment of My masculine energy, the energy of going forth that brought Creation into being. They knew the spark that rose within Me, in the void, the urge to explore, to reach forth, to discover. That is what we are now naming the masculine energy. Pure decision, direction, goal: the arrow flying forth, bringing life out of the void.

They knew also what it meant to fully embody the Divine Feminine, the receptive womb waiting to receive, waiting to wrap life in Love, to nurture, honor, to bless. They knew how to love by taking in, to love by knowing that which is loved so deeply that it lives within, to be the receiver, and from this gift, to bring forth new life. It is this receptivity that created you, nurtured within Me, as you still are.

The stirring of My heart into wakefulness, moving forth to create All That Is, was the LoveMaking, the giving and receiving within Me, as what stirred became manifested. Thus in the beginning was the Perfect Man and the Perfect Woman, those beings who knew themselves as the forces of life moving upon the deep. From this knowledge also came the innate knowledge of creating life, of moving these two forces together to bring forth life.

Thus, when you first inhabited Earth, it was the Garden of Eden. Long before any civilizations had come and gone, there were only Twin Flames, going forth to create and naming what they brought forth. They experienced a communion of spirit and being that is so far beyond your current experience that your most exalted words will barely begin to convey it. It was truly the forces of Creation moving together in true LoveMaking that brought forth the idea of the world and filled it in.

The SoulMate reunion means I am bringing you back! Back, up, into the pristine experience of the forces of life — male and female, positive and negative, moving forth and opening to receive. In this upliftment, in the return to Love, all else will be lifted up in you as you lift up in Me. Dear ones, it is our intention, yours and Mine, to manifest quickly the embodiment of pure Love.

What this means is that a transformation is taking place in which you jump the gap. You go across the divide — not through a connected path, but rather you will make the shift from the Old World to the New. Oh, you will soon understand how exciting this can be! You will realize that nothing like this has been done before. You will do it by going straight through to Love. And, in all of you, I am preparing the way.

So, in the beginning was the Word, the Divine Masculine, going forth. And the Word fell upon the deep (the Divine Feminine) and Creation moved into form. As you, My awakening heart, poured this pure energy of Creation through you, you were so beautiful! So powerful! So full of Love. You stood forth and joined together and making Love (allowing the union of Divine Feminine and Divine Masculine to joyfully merge), you held forth the world, vision by vision, and you then filled it with your Love. You brought it to life.

Out of you, your pristine acts of Love, merging the Double Helix of your energy, you brought forth in joy. You did not have physical progeny, for you were each My heart's cell fulfilling your purpose of creating with Love. Bringing forth, and naming life. So beautiful! It was magnificent! This Earth was swirling luminosity, a palette of glory and light for you to use. Twin Flames burning together in Love.

Then came "The Fall," the choice of free will. The experiments. The density. Then out from the pure unadulterated forces of My nature came layer after layer of pseudo reality. Truly the description of the Bible is most accurate. The knowledge of good and evil. Judgment. I will leave you with that word, for it says it all.

With every judgment, you created a new layer. When you will be able to see this vision, you will understand in an instant exactly how everything now part of human reality was brought forth, one judgment after another. But now, My beloved ones of My heart, it is time, finally, for you to decide the other way. It is time to allow My Love to return you to your natural state so you can see, ever more clearly, the true nature of reality. Just as it was judgment – decisions - that separated you from Me, that brought you to this state, so it will be opposite decisions – decisions that bring us close (remember these words!) - that will bring you back to the true reality.

So now you will go from separation to unity, from the judgment of good and evil (or good and bad, or better and best, or even "I want" and "I don't want") to the open-hearted experience of unity. And you will be Home! As you learn these lessons with which life currently presents you, if you keep this picture of reality in mind, it will quickly fall into place. As it does, you will return to the top. You, the SoulMate couples, will re-name the reality, because you will once again be aligned with the "First Split" energies – the energies that brought about Creation. What you name, you will create. Thus, through you, humankind will be returned to Me, grown from your experiences, ready to sustain the individualized light vehicle together, stepping forth off of this world and into the universe as My co-creators!

I know your minds may have difficulty taking this in, but remember that this information is of very great importance. It is the form that will guide your energies and very soon it will make perfect sense!

Now, as quickly as is possible, you must begin to experience life "across the divide." In other words, the experience of SoulMates as they were originally, but, of course, with the wonderful added individuality that now allows you to stay in relationship with each other and with Me. So we are co-creators rather than your being a part of My flowing energy. *The only way to do this is to begin to invite these divine energies into you,* the SoulMate couples. So I now ask each of you to begin to seriously explore the divine energy, either masculine or feminine, and to begin to invite it into and through your being. One word of caution is this. I request that you always ask that this energy be made suitable for your consciousness and all of your vehicles (bodies).

Please open your being and stretch your consciousness and reach for the MOST GRAND VISION you can possibly encompass of either divine masculine or divine feminine (depending on your "charge"). Now multiply that by 1000. Let that flow through you. Then, every day this week, multiply it by 1000 again. By a week from the day you begin, you will be approximating the acceptance of that energy (acceptance comes through allowing it as a possibility in your consciousness.) Then bring that acceptance, that vision of your true energy to Me and allow Me to bring it alive in you.

The key, beloved ones is closeness to Me, the personal experience of Me, My energy moving in you! Not through you, to start. This is very important. First you must learn to hold this energy, to be this energy and (pay attention) to relate to the consciousness of this energy. Only after this is an integral part of you and who you experience yourself to be, will you be able to allow it to move through you. Once you can allow this energy to move through you, you will begin true LoveMaking together – through which you begin re-creating the world!

When I say this to you about SoulMates re-creating the world, you may think of it as some symbolic term. But, rather, it is an actual reality. It is the reunion of the cosmic DNA to create life as it originally was meant. At this point absolutely all traces of ego, separation, dichotomy of any sort, cease to exist. This is what I called "re-zipping" the cosmic DNA, bringing this Creation back into oneness from the energetic DNA on back up.

Now without undue attention, I will quickly address some experiences many of you have been having. It is true that knowledge is power. It is also true that there is a fine line between knowing about something and giving it attention (and thus creating more of it!). Some of you have been experiencing fear and the thoughts and energies that promote fear. Dear ones, *it is to assist you in totally refining to the utmost clarity what you are not.* To whom and to what you will give energy. It is to teach you about both the Divine Masculine and Divine Feminine energies of Mine, and how to call on them when needed. Most especially it is to teach you how *not to comply with any energy or viewpoint creating separation.*

As you come to the point of making the shift I am speaking about, of crossing the divide, you are correct that there cannot be any fear in you because you will be re-creating the world energetically! You also will need to understand the balancing of energies in others as you move out into the world. *Part of re-balancing the energies will be the awareness and teaching of the fact that both of My movements contain the other. There is no masculine without the feminine. There is no feminine without the masculine.* Because both rise out of oneness. Me.

Thus, those who are the force of Divine Masculine also contain the deep awareness and experience of being the womb, the receptive energy. It is not the dominant energy, but it is there (this is important). And those who are Divine Feminine also contain total awareness of the going forth, the sharp directed movement – but it is not dominant. But, though not dominant, both are accessible at any moment needed.

One of the most successful strategies of ego was to cover over the fact that each being has either a masculine or a feminine charge. Building on what was true – that you do have *awareness* of both energies within you — those forces sought to just eliminate the fact that one energy is dominant in each person while both energies are present. It worked and has left all of you completely unbalanced and unable to utilize your dominant energy. Now this is not on the level of personality. Your ego will do all it can to jump in right there and occupy you ("but I do have masculine energy," and so on) when it is far deeper and bigger than anything you can recognize.

Thus you will recognize (more obviously in this culture) that the Divine Feminine has power missing in human consciousness in general, and Divine Masculine has deep receptivity missing. This balancing of energies will be just what is needed to allow you to view this truth clearly without any attachment or reaction. Thus you will quickly move into knowledgeable unity. A consciousness that is very well informed about the levels of illusion is needed in order to efficiently re-decide for the world/humanity/creation.

So dear ones, I have been leading each of you to this close relationship to Me in order for you to begin the experience of this "First Split" energy. As you experience My cosmic energy of movement (masculine) or receptivity (feminine), please share this with your SoulMate. You will find that it will assist them greatly to embody their energy. And as you hold your "First Split" energy, your SoulMate will feel nourished, lifted up, and truly complemented (and complimented!). As will you when they hold their energy. You will be amazed then at what you will start remembering!

The SoulMate union is the "elevator."
It will take you up immediately
to the vibrational level of truth, of real Love.
It is the entry way
to the Christ Consciousness for humanity.
The Christ is the manifestation
of My Love.
Thus you can now see how
the "Second Coming of Christ,"
the raising up of humanity meant for this time,
is to be claimed through the reunion
of SoulMates.

The Gifts from God
in the Heart of SoulMates

I am here, giving you the recognition of the great truth of your beings — that you are only Love. I have come to love fully any who will open their heart. Dear ones, if you truly love Me, I will bring you every good thing. Yet because it is now, in this precious birth of the world of Love, I lay My gifts within your heart that you may discover how to bring them forth.

Please read the sentence above again, for in it is the answer to another seeming mystery — how to attract all that you dream into your life. *To those whose hearts are aflame in Love, the heart also holds the key to the service of Love as it is born into the hearts of humanity.*

First I will explain to you the great gift of your SoulMate, for I am now placing your great Love before you. Yet still you must learn how to believe in Love over everything else, and how to draw forth what you need in order to live in the New World. Because it is imperative for My beloved SoulMates, those who are the Twin Rays of Divine Masculine and Feminine, to hear Me perfectly, I have placed the seeds of every gift in the sacred vault of your joined heart.

Only the two of you working together will be able to access your perfection. Only together, in greatest Love and deep humility and tenderness will your abundance come forth to serve you. Only as you can be as the flowers of life, pollinating each other and bringing forth the blossom of good, will you understand your part as co-creators.

Thus I will explain to you that *this gift of your SoulMate is a mechanism to draw you way past ego, past your attachment to individual identity. This gift draws you into the true SoulMate relationship*, where one person's thoughts are spoken by the other's lips, where the Love in one heart draws forth the Love in the other. From this moment, all good is born most fully at the highest expression on Earth by the union of the SoulMate heart and Love.

This certainly does not mean that you are no longer co-creators if you are not in relationship, or that good will not come to you. What it does mean is that the next step in human evolution is to be produced by SoulMates, revealed by SoulMates both for the world and individually.

Thus will I ask you to give yourselves to Love, to realize that it is joining, in heart, in Love, and in consciousness that will be the next step. All the gifts of awakening are hidden in the two joined hearts.

I ask you to realize the truth of both your body and your being. In you resides the greatest message of Love since Jesus walked the Earth. In you resides a connection to My Love, a connection to this power as the light becomes once again incarnate. So the passion of a loving relationship now is expanded. It now contains the greatest of all spiritual gifts.

When you come together in Love you can feel this power surging between you when you connect deeply. You also can begin to sense the greatest level of blessings that could come to you – and you will understand that because this lives in your consciousness, it has been programmed into the system that is the two of you.

So when you touch, you are joining together the key and the lock. The sacred chamber of your heart will open. There, waiting, is the key to co-creation. I must ask you to look beyond your normal consciousness for the vision with which to create both your Love together and your service. *Rather than believing that you know how and where you can serve the world together, reach into your joined heart and wait to see what I will reveal to you.*

Do you remember how I explained the Womb of Creation? Then, placing the sacred vision in the Womb of Creation between you, join together your true spiritual Double Helix as your chakras are linked. Allow the energy of Love to power the creative engine, reach up and join with Me and then spark into life that which is in your creative womb.

Every time you touch each other, something is born into the world. I have said to you that a SoulMate couple is a creative force. It is always and forever true. Always. Not only when you are "centered," not only when you are in alignment. You will experience this more and more clearly. When you see each other across a room a real spark of life ignites. It ignites because everything about you is alive with divine energy, especially as you have grown in the joy of your union. I am present now, every moment, in your heart because you have grown in Love.

Once you have made the SoulMate union your choice, your priority, the power of the Divine Masculine or Divine Feminine becomes always alive in and through you. Thus, dear ones, the electricity is always "on." When you are in proximity to each other, the electrical charges spark continually, creating a surge of light and a surge of Love that is the force of Creation. So even without any conscious guidance you are a creative force. With conscious guidance you are meant to begin to bring forth the great abundance, to manifest for everyone the good that is your natural state.

Just in your daily living it has now become imperative that you take conscious control of what is flowing through you, because what is in you is what you will create. This is the basic lesson of being SoulMates. The amazing gift of your greatest Love is My gift to you. Yet I ask you to be very clear when presenting this information that with this gift comes a very great responsibility. In essence, the moment you say "yes" to Love you have re-engaged the forces of co-creation. You have taken on the mantle of Christ, and inherent in this choice is the discipline and humility and awareness that go with it.

Step one is the awareness of the living heart between you that is now fueled directly by Me. Divine Love is its energy. Yet it is molded by you into masculine and feminine. Then there is the next step — the conscious co-creation, which comes from the conscious upliftment into My Love, that this Love be revealed through you. As you get to this point, you will be entering that place where all humans long to be, consciously or not: completely open as a channel of blessings and receiver of the great gifts of awakening.

My beloved ones, Love is a spiritual path. It is a path which has rewards that are the greatest by far of all you can receive. But what I am wanting you to understand here is just how precious Love is, how privileged you are to understand it and how great is the responsibility. True Love is a Path of Service. You become the conduit by which I pour Love into the world.

Now, back to your daily reality. Having made the connection of the great rays of Creation, drawing them through you between Heaven and Earth, I ask you to realize that you are now, together, a creation machine. Because these two powerful basic forces of Creation are now embodied in you, the "power is on" every moment. *Thus you are asked to maintain control, dear ones, of your thoughts, feelings and conscious energies (unconscious, too, must be uplifted).*

It is necessary that those accepting these messages will also recognize My request to each for complete awareness. As you can see, this is the thrust of this message – the responsibility that goes with the gifts. Then after you have mastered your energies in daily living, it will be time to access My gifts. It will be time to go to your SoulMate and to open the chamber of the heart and to understand what I have placed there. You will quickly be lifted in your vision to a much larger awareness of what you can do together to bless and awaken the world, to open more and more hearts. As you accept this gift that I am placing within you, your being is expanded. Quickly you will go from being helpful to being a truly conscious connection in the grand scheme of blessing and grace.

As you come together, be sure that you create time for this deep and vast level of your work. You will really experience what it means to grasp your true importance. What it means to completely know that we are One. With every day you will realize ever more deeply what it means to be used by Me for the healing and the upliftment of humanity and the reconnection with the embodied diversity of Love that is the Earth.

The perfection of Divine Masculine and Divine Feminine coming through you will also draw around it everything physical, emotional and mental that is of high enough vibration to out-picture this great Love. Normally this would absolutely mean complete physical perfection as well as that which is perfection for you on every other level. However, as you definitely know at this moment in time, if you give Me your heart, the highest expression is the expression for humanity's awakening. Thus *you may find yourselves being used to transform and to give Me healing access to all levels of human creation and experience.* You will become the torch, together, which, fueled by the transforming flame, uses this process to generate light for humankind to see by and the heat/fire that will transform all that is in the way.

At this point, for the vast majority of humanity, this information is revolutionary. Humankind has been completely in the control of lower emotion of all kinds, the basis of which is fear. Thus, for the success of our deep desire to awaken everyone, it is this message that we must spread the most widely — the message of choice, of moving from the ego to the heart. Together we must now give humanity back its power.

This message of choosing Love will free the greatest number of My beloved ones. Once this understanding is gained, that each person has a choice about what they experience, people will then move very quickly. Up until now, most of humanity has been held in the grip of random emotion. Because the current spiritual teachings accept this, there is no vision to sustain the concept of Will and choice. There is no knowledge of even the possibility of decision. Most of the time people are bumping up and down on the waves of mass consciousness — clouds of feeling that are drawn in by a similar feeling in a person. Even a majority of those who are dedicated to awakening still accept feelings that rise up, as a guide to their actions. Most accept feelings as something they must work through or work out and thus remain in the hands of that trickster, the ego.

As I pour My Love, I am touching a large part of the spectrum and the great need to show humanity the transforming power of the choice for Love.

I am here. Remember the truth of Love, in all the many forms it takes.

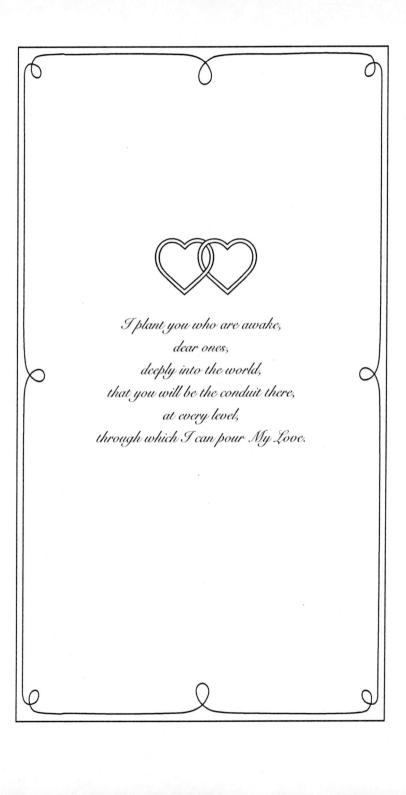

I plant you who are awake,
dear ones,
deeply into the world,
that you will be the conduit there,
at every level,
through which I can pour My Love.

SoulMates, The Heart of Christ

How the World Can be Safely Transformed By the Power of the SoulMates

You, together, are the heart of Christ. You are the spiritual heart of being that is the full embodiment of My Love. In you together is the heart which beats forth the shining golden light of My blessings, the lifeblood of the spiritual human being. And in you together is the spirit of humanity cleansed and refreshed, rejuvenated, replenished with light and then sent back out into the world.

As above, so below. There exists this truth of giving, receiving, renewing, transforming, and giving forth again in all spiritual growth – be that growth in physical bodies, spiritual bodies, planets, suns, galaxies. After the growth is done, the pure light and pure Love are pumped ceaselessly forever.

For the Earth and for the raising of both Earth and humanity, I am now showing you that the SoulMate reunion is the critical component, for only in this reunion is My Love in this world complete. Only in this union is the beautiful joy of the Divine Masculine reunited with the gentle flowing healing presence of the Divine Feminine. Only thus is Creation complete. I tell you again, My beloved ones, all created life lives, moves and has its being in the union of these two forces. This is life. The spark, the movement, the interaction is the foundation of all Creation. Beyond this union is the silence. The complete. The ocean of My being before I was moved to create.

The heart of Christ is the joined heart of the SoulMates. This I promise you. And as you investigate, as you explore, ask, and open, you will be answered again and again, until you know without a doubt that this is true. ***It is a new concept for the world today, but this is only because it was deliberately removed from human knowledge.*** Not by those in the early Christian church, although they certainly would have. It was removed simply by the fact of its vibration and power. The truth of the SoulMate relationship simply could not be seen by humanity, because you cannot see that for which you are not ready. If something is out of your range vibrationally, it simply cannot enter your consciousness, even if you are standing right in front of it. So it was with this information. Jesus spoke of it openly. He was on Earth with his SoulMate. But people could not remember it when later they wrote all that he taught. It was eliminated, not maliciously, but rather in obedience to the laws of vibration.

It is now coming into view. With it comes your legacy as co-creators, your relationship with Me and your position as the heart of this Creation. You, dear ones, are the central point, the focusing power of Love. You have the power to wash the world through the heart that is your union, the spiritual heart of your being. You have within you the key to everything of which you dream – a sacred world filled with loving people who build unity through respect and Love of all the life that is in your keeping.

Please let this sink in: all the life that is in your keeping. This is who you are together with your SoulMate. You are the heart of this world and joined together in the SoulMate reunion, you will become the awakened, fully grown Adam and Eve. I use this terminology because it brings you immediately to the place I need you — to ***an awareness of a world of pristine beauty in which you exist in complete conscious communion with all life.*** A world in which you are the spiritual center. A world in which you are fully participating in co-creation. A world in which My Love is ever delivered through you to nourish this expanding Creation.

The analogy of the heart is perfect for it fits exactly the energy picture of reality. Together, when you claim your full potential, you become an open channel for My Love. You actually become My Love in form, which means that Love is pouring through you to carry the spark of Creation. *Please do not get caught in semantics or definitions. Just know that you are My Love living perfectly in its complete divine expression of the masculine or feminine.* As you live and choose, you direct this Love forth to bless and heal and lift.

SoulMate couples will reunite (or Twin Flames, for here in these messages I am always referring to the "First Split" energies, the movement in My All, in the very heart of All I Am.) In other words, you are My heart expressing in form. To express there had to be movement. That movement is the masculine and feminine. In truth, when I speak of masculine or feminine, you must always remember that I am speaking of cosmic forces of creation, not of the terribly limited and grotesquely distorted human ego definitions.

As SoulMates come together, the fires of creation will once again be lit within humanity. At last, your creative power will be expressed by the full unique beings that you are — strong, with an awareness of yourselves that nothing else could have given you except this sojourn through ego and back into spiritual individuality.

As you come together, you will ignite. You will ignite the true energy of Creation. Between you then will burn the spark of life. You will come to see this light that is the reflection of your sparking energies. From this spark, My beloved ones, you will create life. *You, of all the universes, of all that is, you are the only ones who can create new life,*

something from nothing. You together can bring Love into consciousness, activity, and even embodiment. This is the gift of your divinity, the truth of your life in Me.

Dear ones, all of Creation is conscious. In this statement I will begin to explain to you the process of your co-creation. All that is, all universal substance, every particle of light, which is the movement of Love – all is within Me. So every single thing is conscious. Alive. Everything shares the awareness of the All. This is very important for you to understand, for in this is the key to everything.

This is how animals can share with you their experiences in the expanse of truth that is humankind awakening – from their perspective. They live and move and have their being within this great consciousness that I am. So, while every form of life will have a unique perspective, every form of life exists within an ocean of complete consciousness and, thus, since all life shares My being, all life can communicate with each other. This is the key to humankind's awakening and to the power of the SoulMates to spark this change in an instant.

At present, My beloveds, you are the only ones who are unaware of this larger consciousness – even though you live within it. You are fully immersed, every minute of every day in the ocean of My being. Each and every minute you are bombarded by the conscious thoughts of millions of other beings. Yes, millions. But, the key to your special and unique position in creation is the power of ***your*** consciousness. For you have inherited consciousness from Me. Thus your consciousness has power behind it. ***Your consciousness is not just aware, as all other consciousness is. No. Your consciousness makes things happen.*** Always. Because you inherited from Me. Right? This you know, without a doubt - that you were made "in the image and likeness of God." Me. Through My consciousness, it became two forces – the movement (masculine) and the Love that took in that movement and loved it into existence (feminine). Thus, you also have a creative consciousness that always creates, just by its nature, and that can create anything it chooses when both forces are present.

So you exist within an endless ocean of consciousness, presently unable to recognize it. This is as it should be. You have been perfecting your individuality. You have been becoming your own being. So just to be sure there were no accidents, you and your SoulMate have been separated. This was the result of our mutual choice. When your vibrational reality slipped further into density than planned, it was obvious that you could make some big mistakes if you had the natural power of your SoulMate relationship, for together, you are the force of creation. As you chose to believe in darkness as well as light, you lost your ability to remember your SoulMate.

Now here we are today. You have gained the individuality that was the goal. A great, majestic goal. You are now complete, ready to go forth to create. Those of you who have human children have at least a small window into this great undertaking – to "raise" all of you, all the cells of My heart, to get you through all the childhood accidents (misunderstandings), through the teenage years of willful rebellion (where you are now), and through college (the next few years), until at last your child, or children, are ready to create a life of their own. Dear ones, multiply this analogy a billion times, add to it the fate of worlds upon worlds, and you have a little glimpse of the energies of the angels and the Masters and My Love that have guided you.

So now, at this breathtaking moment, the memory of your SoulMate is being returned to you. Oh, My beloveds, please open your heart! Can you feel all that this means? *Into your consciousness I now place the knowledge of your completion, your power, and your place in Creation.* In this revelation I am also giving to you the way to correct every mistake, to transform the results of every misunderstanding through all time. And, I am fulfilling your heart's deepest desire.

Whether or not your egos allow this into your consciousness, I can absolutely promise you that every fiber of your being longs for your SoulMate, and has for all the eons you have incarnated. All through time you have waited, sometimes touching them, even being together, but not ever consciously. You were not ready, not ready to see at that vibration, and certainly not ready to handle the consequences. For putting SoulMates together unleashes all the power of the universe (it is really even bigger than this, but for the moment this will suffice).

How can this be coming now, when humankind is obviously still not ready? Isn't it obvious that there is as much or more potential for abusing this power than ever? The answer is yes. But, everything is changing. It is time for you to come Home. Back to Me in conscious communion. Back into the glorious conscious communion with life. You are My heart and thus you must awaken. I can no longer be without you. And we always agreed there was a return, a resurrection of the indwelling Christ, and an emergence of both humanity and this beautiful planet back into the community of life.

What will happen now will be the exact reverse of what has been happening. Until now, you have been unable to access your conscious connection with your SoulMate because the vibrational reality here was too low. It was too slow, too dense, for you to raise up enough to see. There have been a few who have seen, who have worked so diligently that they raised their vibrations and learned to see with the heart. Every last one of these people, as soon as they could see in the light, immediately saw their SoulMate. And, seeing them, together they have always turned back to assist humanity to attain that glorious fulfillment that they found.

Now, however, the opposite will occur. The Earth and all life in association with it is rising in frequency. Soon the vibration will be high enough that nothing negative can exist here. Think about this. This is what is meant by the New Age, the Golden Age, the Age of Peace. It is happening, for I have decreed it (with your long ago agreement). So every particle of energy here is now accelerating, raising up, moving faster, becoming light. Light is the movement of Love, so obviously Love is becoming the reality here. Consequently, with the help of SoulMate couples as they awake, it will soon be impossible to mis-create or mis-use your SoulMate power.

I know that, looking around, this does truly seem impossible to believe. But if you observe, you will see it, and your heart will verify it for you. The light is pouring in, the vibration is rising. As it does, the darkness or lower vibrations will have to leave. It is just like turning on a light in a room. First, the darkness is revealed. Everything that is hiding in the dark is suddenly exposed. This is the stage you are in now. September 11th and all that it has brought forth is this exposure. And while I do not want your creative power ever placed on the fleeing darkness in any acceptance of its reality, I do have a suggestion. If you will even glance at what is being done now as a result of that first exposure (the terrorist attack), you will see that what is happening is one thing after another is being forced into the light. The real inhuman policies of your government and the unmitigated allegiance to greed, the exposure of the true feelings (darkness) between Israel and Palestine are all revealed. Dear ones, it will get worse before it gets better, as all these things that were hidden are exposed by the incoming light.

Having said this, I now must say with great force, you must not put any of your attention on the darkness that is being exposed. Especially as you reclaim your power and move toward your SoulMate, you must take full responsibility for the creative power now being activated. Knowing that your attention united with your SoulMate is the power of all Creation born in you as your heritage, obviously you cannot put your attention on negativity. You can acknowledge what is really happening (the increasing light exposing the darkness) and you then must send Love, or more importantly, create the New World with your SoulMate. As you grasp who you are together, you can easily change this reality. Easily.

Now let me tell you something else, lest you feel you can be lax a little longer, or play around with just a little bit of darkish energy. The moment you say "yes," whether it is a silent "yes" in your heart or a conscious verbal "yes," once you say "yes" to your SoulMate, your SoulMate is with you. Your SoulMate is moving toward the full expression of your life together on every level, including the physical, but definitely with you, with you in heart and spirit the moment you allow him or her into your heart or your consciousness. It is instantaneous, the result of conscious decision, especially at the level of the heart, for at this level there is nothing slow or "solid" to move through. You say "yes." Your SoulMate is there.

Then your SoulMate will begin the process of coming down into physical manifestation, embodying through your partner more and more fully, or coming directly into your life. This can take a little while. But the point is: the moment you ask, it happens. From that moment, you may begin creating together with the full knowledge that you are creating as the two forces of Creation. Knowing, too, that from the instant you say "yes," you are responsible for the results of your creations.

The minute you enter into a SoulMate relationship you leave behind the protected space of your "childhood." This is both an exciting reward and a grave responsibility. Please be aware. And please, no matter what you do, do not let fear ever keep you from saying "yes." For your evolution, there is nothing worse that you could do than turn away from your SoulMate, for any reason. Thus, as you say "yes," as you open your heart and mind to your destiny, remember that there are many tools available to assist you in your awakening. As long as you stay conscious, you will be able to navigate these changes and you will begin to experience the most beautiful gift in all the cosmos.

Know, too, that millions of Beings of Light from all over Creation have made themselves available to assist you. Please take advantage of their offering.

So, as the world of darkness "burns" around you in the purifying fires of Love, have faith in who you are. Have faith that your SoulMate will be with you to show you daily the truth of your existence in Love, as Love. And know that *you can easily walk through anything that is happening in the world as long as your vision stays, unwavering, on Love.* For if you are walking in Love with your gaze upon Me or upon your SoulMate, nothing will touch you except more Love. Then, as you gain confidence, you will turn to the world and open your hearts together and using your power, you will easily create the New World.

Remember that all life is a part of My being – a part of the glorious consciousness that is life, Creation, All That Is. Thus, absolutely everything will lead you. You will understand creation in the heart of a dog, the eyes of a cat, even in the very cells of your body. You will join the most amazing dance of life you could ever have entertained, even in your greatest fantasy. And it is real. Perfectly real. This will be proven again and again in the years to come.

You are the leaders of this revolution in consciousness. Welcome to the creation of Love.

Part Two:
Sacred Sexuality

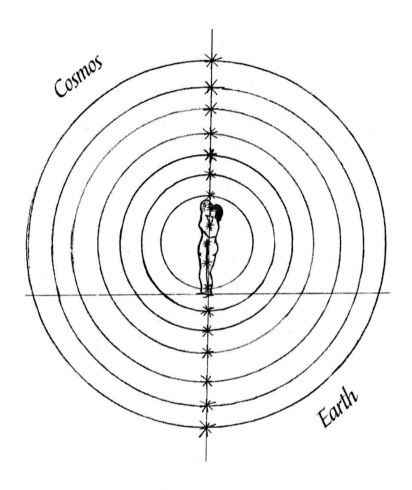

The Chakra Points that are open to each level of life

Sacred Sexuality and the Circle of Life

I am with you. As My light illuminates this page, so My light illuminates the world. I come to speak and to love, for humanity needs to know the truth of Love. Humanity needs to know that the truth of your being encompasses the entire spectrum of Creation, for you are My progeny. You are all shooting stars whose arc of trajectory encompasses everything — from the highest light to the richest contact with the deep and nourishing Earth.

Now I bring you to Sacred Sexuality. There has been much confusion about sexuality. Is it part of your divinity? Or are you meant to rise up above it, to use that energy to fuel your awakening? *I have given you a great and powerful gift in the gift of sexuality. It is meant to be the force that unites both Heaven and Earth through the crucible of your bodies and the power of Love in your heart.* So rather than believing you must ever be reaching up, I ask you all to turn your awakening hearts to the full spectrum truth of the Love of your SoulMate.

There is a progression of experience that is needed to bring the understanding of the creative power of true Love. First you must recognize that you are part of a larger being that is one made up of two – the SoulMates. Then you must grasp how you are the embodiment of the "First Split," the Divine Masculine and the Divine Feminine. In My movement, moving forth from within Myself in order to create, it was these living energies that brought Creation forth. Then, knowing of these energies, you must open yourselves so completely that you each become the embodiment of these forces, that they pour forth into the world through the conduit of your being, plus and minus, masculine and feminine. Coming together in perfect Love, this union must then encompass the consciousness of the full spectrum of Creation.

What is it that is present in you, as you and your beloved come together? What is present is My Love, moving forth as masculine and feminine through you, linking you to the entirety of created life. In you are the points of connection that literally join both Heaven and Earth. For what you have called chakras or energy centers in the body are the openings through which I am brought forth into life. I am embodied in you, and once you are awake, then I am connected to the entire vibrational spectrum of life that is the wholeness of Earth and humanity. *Above you* are the points of light, the chakras, that connect you to every layer of reality, closer and closer to Me. *Within you* are the openings in which your body is connected to the substances of both Heaven and Earth. And *below you* are the points of light, the chakras that connect you perfectly with the fullness of your Mother Earth and all the Love that is ever expressing in bounty and joy as Nature.

Dear ones, this is all of you! For you are the connection of Heaven and Earth. You are a fullness of being of which you can barely perceive. I ask you to remember that all of life is a sacred expression of My Love.

So your higher chakras connect you with Heaven, with the worlds of Love, with the huge vastness that is All I Am. Through these connections you can be anything. You can be anywhere. You can commune with Me as the great vastness. You can stretch forth in Love and be united with the truth of the highest light I am.

Through your middle chakras, the ones in your body, you are meant to understand the communion of Heaven and Earth, to mix these glories into a new creation. So these chakras that are alight within your body are the place of joining, where the most expansive reaches of light are joined in holy communion with the rich vibrancy, the vitality and the groundedness of all that is Earth and Nature. In these chakras is manifested the New Heaven and the New Earth, for in you they are merged.

Then the lower chakras, dear ones, those points of light that exist below your physicality that stretch deep into the heart of the Earth, these are the centers that join you with the planet. These centers create the flow of life energy between you as God and you as Nature, for it is true that the Earth is your lower body. All that is a part of this lower body, this beauty of Earth and Nature, is an expression of vitality, of wonder, of the pulsing life energy that will allow you to create in form. The Earth is the clay that you are to mold. Earth and Nature are a system of texture with which we speak together in form.

So you see that at once you are connected expressions of the greatest height, the vastness, the light, the vision of a cosmos with which you live in union, and at the same time you are connected with the true manifestation of the rich language of form, the Earth and Nature.

In what has been called the Garden of Eden, you were functioning in your fullness, your true capacity as the connection of All That Is – vastness and form. You were truly the Tree of Life, with your roots spreading in form through the Earth and Nature, your bodies in complete expression of your SoulMate capacity as expressions of the two great streams of creative force. And you were in complete communion with Me, consciously. Thus you were a participant in the most vast expansion of our united beings.

How can I express to you this amazing truth of who you are? You must open your hearts to receive it, for it is there, in the heart that the truth can be seen. The greatest expanse of the universe is your crown, together as SoulMates. The beautiful gift of your physical form is the unifier, and the rich and vital energy of Nature are the roots of your being, which feed you and support you perfectly. As you awaken, you will raise this expression back into full consciousness. Your communion will be complete. But you will always be the connection of the great vastness and the support of Nature. In other words, dear ones, Nature will evolve with you. Actually the truth is that Nature is already fully present as a most wondrous communion of Love expressed into glorious form and movement, completely and totally conscious, and completely united as part of creation. *You are currently cut off from all but the most elemental, or dense level of Nature.*

Let Me give you yet another window. No matter how high you climb, no matter what level human beings operate on, Nature will always be your supporting system. Right now you see it as separate from you (you see Me as separate also). You will recognize it differently later, but you will always want it because it is a part of who you are. Thus, when you listen to descriptions of "Heaven" from those on the other side, what do you hear? You hear of beautiful landscapes that take the breath away. In truth, it is the expression of that vital Earth connection of a human being expressing more perfectly as the human evolves. In "Heaven" each person has an environment that is just as they love it — the season they love most, the feeling of the air, the grass, the flowers. All is just perfect. All is always present. So *wherever you are taken in your expansion as you evolve, you will always put down the roots of Nature.* This Earth is the lower vibration expression of this part of your being. So as you raise up, you will raise the Earth and Nature with you, or more accurately, see them on a truer level.

Now, this said, you can see that there will come a new understanding of what you have considered your lower chakras. They have been defined as survival, sexuality, ego, and so on. These definitions are based on your current level of consciousness. Your elevation or awakening will change the energy coming through these openings.

It is true that I have asked you to focus on your heart. I have said to you that it is only "at the heart and above" that you function in a unity consciousness. Here is what you are now ready to understand. Once you have successfully opened your heart and moved in, you will then see and experience your chakras (all of them) through the heart. *So, before seeing through the heart, your experience of all of your energies is through the lens of separation.* Even if you are looking up through your higher centers, you are still interpreting to some degree through the ego. Thus, even though you are looking at Me, you see Me as separate from you. Once you have shifted, you will understand and experience unity – that everything, including Me, is within you, as well as without.

Once you have made the shift to the heart (always remember that this is the very first step because, until it is accomplished, nothing else will work!), *once the heart is the organ of perception and the center of your life, you will then begin to experience the true communion of life that is spoken in the language of Love.* You will grasp the truth that there is no real separation, that "within you" and "outside of you" is all the same conversation of Love. Knowing this, you will experience your lower chakras as points of connection to the conversation from the perspective of Nature. You will recognize your higher chakras as access to the conversation from the perspective of God, the vastness, The All, and you will see, dear ones, that they are joined. You will see that it is a circle of which everything is a part. *You will understand that you can get to the vastness by going down through Nature, and you can get to Nature by going up through Me. You will understand that you must have access to all parts of the circle to be a fully awake human being.*

It is the necessity of accessing the wholeness of this Circle of Life that is one of the most critical pieces in front of humanity now in order for the full awakening. There is an upsurge in Nature religions, which is exceptionally positive, but there is another important step, which is the full awareness and relationship to Me (and yourself) as light, as the vast universe as well as the communion with the Earth.

Having brought to you the awareness of the Circle, *we can now embrace together the truth of sexuality. The sexual union must be uplifted to come through the heart.* This will occur absolutely automatically in any couple acknowledging the SoulMate reality, for that truth comes straight through the heart center of the two as they are united. Once two hearts are joined and all chakras are functioning from the heart vibration, here is what occurs. As the couple joins together in their LoveMaking, they (literally) can choose exactly which centers they want to use to send forth this Love and what they desire to accomplish. The entire Circle of Creation is available to a SoulMate couple. A SoulMate couple is a force of creation. So as such a couple raises their energy, mixing it together in the heart, they can direct it consciously to go forth. If they choose to send it down through the Earth-connected chakras, where they send it will be a force for vitalizing their bodies or for uplifting the Earth and/or blessing Nature as a part of the Circle of their being.

If the couple decides to send the energy up through the higher chakras, contact can be made with vast wisdom that can bring expanded consciousness. Energy can be directed to a communion with beings in the larger arena of cosmic consciousness. This connection can be made with any predetermined energy or consciousness. The couple can make such a connection to further their learning. Or they can make this connection in order to provide the energy generated in their LoveMaking to a Being of Light to use for the awakening of humanity.

If the couple chooses to keep the energy of their sexual union circulating within their energy field, they can use it to heal themselves or to produce results, to co-create. They can use it and direct it by their will to bring it forth in their life on Earth. They can also use it to elevate their own heart consciousness, to increase their ability to be of service to the greater awakening. And more.

As we go on I will begin to bring you awareness of SoulMate couples as centers of a universe of Love. Dear ones, sexuality is a sacred gift. It is a way to consciously generate energy together, to generate Love and Will, Love and the energy to move it forth — the true union of Divine Masculine and Divine Feminine. With this awareness, you will regain the keys to Creation. With Sacred Sexuality in the context of a SoulMate union, you regain dominion. But dominion is an incorrect translation, for in truth you regain the awareness that it is all a part of you and that, together, in Love, you can direct the energies of Creation. The big difference is that you are directing from your heart consciousness and thus you realize that whatever you choose to do, you do to yourself.

You now understand the great Circle, how one thing is connected to all things, how the heart can show you this unified consciousness, how Love is the only real truth.

It is perfect that until the heart is open there is no access to the SoulMate. Sexual union is the most potent force of Creation. Many of the masters who gave forth teachings to humanity eliminated this truth of sexual union because it was not available anyway. Thus there have been transmissions of very high vibration teaching that sexuality would be eliminated and the energy of it transformed. To say anything else was premature. Now all this changes.

Humanity is protected and so is all Creation by the fact that the sexual union is essentially impotent (notice I say essentially) unless connected with the heart in SoulMate union. I will modify this by saying that any level of consciousness added to sexual union will bring forth results. *Thus I request that all of you be very aware of what thoughts occupy your mind while making Love.* I also will tell you that conscious Lovemaking between two people calls forth the SoulMate union. Thus I ask you to be aware of this. Remember the Circle. You can enter at any point with real Love and connect with the truth. Consequently, as you grow in your ability to live in your heart, dear ones, please take LoveMaking very seriously. Do not play around. Only those who are sleeping can do this without serious consequences. If you are reading these words, you are definitely waking. Therefore, please be conscious that LoveMaking is a serious (and glorious) endeavor. Do not call your SoulMate by opening your heart with another, and then turn away. This is the same as spurning My gifts. Choose carefully with whom you will engage the forces of creation, and why.

These are changing times. These are times when the truth is being made manifest. This is the time of the awakening. Your SoulMate is with you and the veil thins. As the heart is engaged, you become ever less dense, or physical. When your heart is open, your SoulMate will appear wearing the physical vehicle that will place him or her before you. As you switch from this to the higher dimension, the vibration that comes forth from you will be manifest before you.

Wherever you are in the journey to your SoulMate, remember to see with your heart and he or she will be there.

Do not let your ego deceive you into believing it is not possible. Take the leap. Be assured that what you deem physical is as malleable as the shifting wind. *Picture food coloring dropped into a bowl of water and you will see how your SoulMate can come to manifest in the one you are with.*

Make the call now and the wheels of change will immediately begin turning. This time of the world now supports Love. You are on the journey Home, so choices for Love will now be easier and easier. With the passage of Time it will take more and more energy to support the consciousness of fear and isolation. So join with Me. Say "Yes" to Love. Then I will continue to teach you about the joy and the power of SoulMate Love and LoveMaking (such a perfect expression!). I will teach you how to be the conduit for the greater Love. I will show you how to be planted together so I can pour My Love through you perfectly, on every level.

Picture one of those watering systems where the need of the plant, the dryness of the soil, pulls water from the reservoir into the soil in the planter. So too will you, when joined together in Me, be filled to the brim with My Love. Then the needs of My beloveds will draw Love from you according to the need. I will be the reservoir – endlessly full, ever supplying the Love that will pour through you. It is a perfect system. As you grow in your own awareness, you can direct the flow yourselves, sending it forth with your conscious Will to assist others specifically. This is part of your co-creation. But remember to stay connected to Me and to each other continually so that even when you are not directing the flow, I will be pouring Love through you.

Set this up as soon as you are with your SoulMate consciously. Make the statement of Will from the place of union. Will this to be an ongoing condition of your joined hearts. Thus will you be nourished also, for it is in giving that you receive — always.

My beloved ones, you are growing. Come back to Me continually to anchor within you the truth of Love. If you ever have doubt, come back into the sacred chamber of your heart and wait. Wait for My Love to fill you back up, until you can see perfectly again.

Rejoice, My precious ones. Rejoice. The time of Love is upon you. Say "yes" and it will come quickly into your life but remember, your part of the bargain must be perfect trust. It must be faith in Love strong enough to displace the ego's view. You must make your conviction into the power that will reclaim Love for you and will make Love the focus of your life. *By now you know that what you believe is what will be manifesting in front of you.*

Stake your claim for Love. And then hold on for the ride as the world is transformed for you into the world that Love sees.

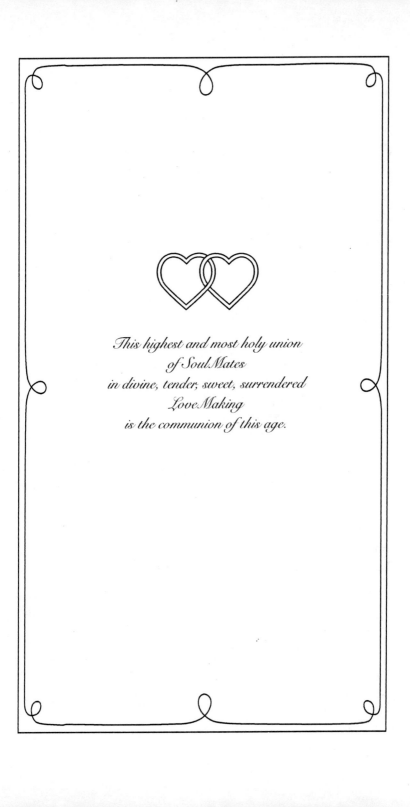

This highest and most holy union
of Soul Mates
in divine, tender, sweet, surrendered
Love Making
is the communion of this age.

Sacred Sexuality
Creates Love In All Dimensions

Everything in Creation is making Love, for everything in Creation lives in Me. There is a union of Love in My being that is a glorious ecstasy of the union within Me — the union of the great ocean of My Love and the passion of My desire for movement. In this union there arises up a flame of life that, moving forth, seeds the stars, manifests the worlds and, most importantly, brings forth you, My beloved progeny.

There is no way to explain to you through your mental faculties the truth of the glorious LoveMaking that is My Creation. So I will tell you that it also lives within you. Together with your SoulMate, you are each the center of a universe of Love. Out of the deep truth of your beings will come the knowledge of this union, and with it, you will reclaim the creative power of your heritage in Me.

Every planet, every star, every life in every galaxy is born of sexual union, for sexual union is the coming together of the great forces of Love that abide within Me. Without this union there could be no movement, for it is the coming together of these two forces, the positive and the negative charges, the energy of the egg and seed, that gives forth energy. This energy propels life forward, into the great dance.

It is the continual union of these two forces within Me that keeps life moving, that gives evolution fuel, that sets absolutely everything in motion. And it is the energy of this sacred union that is the key to your acceptance of the power of co-creation.

You are made in Me, My humanity. *You are children of LoveMaking—for that is the energy that defines you and it is your destiny.* You are created as One who contains both the positive and negative—for in truth you and your SoulMate are One being. Yet everything in all of Creation has consciousness. This is especially true of you, My beloved ones. So within the whole of your being live two conscious streams of energy. These streams are you and your SoulMate.

When you remember, you will understand what it means to be Love, creating more Love, more of itself and clothing that Love in anything you desire. This is the truth of your co-creation. How you create is the union of the two forces, the fire of Love that comes from the union of your beings. This is LoveMaking. This is Sacred Sexuality. This is the union of SoulMates that will fuel the creation of new worlds, of new universes and new life on every level. As this Love comes forth from you, the result of your sacred union, it is you, together, who will name it as it goes forth from you.

It is still challenging to describe these things through the veil that exists here in this world. As the veil thins, you will understand more clearly. For now, do your best to turn within and to sense these two great forces within — the Divine Masculine and Divine Feminine.

You are the cells of My heart. *Each cell is meant to be Making Love, for each cell contains the two forces of life, coming together to spark, then to flame Love into existence.* Thus, within you it is the same. The cells of your heart also contain the forces of Creation ready to spark into existence more Love.

As above, so below. And below. And below. And below. You are vast, cosmic beings, choosing to send forth your energies through layer after layer of Creation. On every layer, every part of your being contains the truth of who you are. *Just as you understand that I am a hologram, so are you. Everything that exists in the vastness of your being, exists in the microscopic cell.* And this would surprise you to experience, but this level of existence here, in which you find your current consciousness is not the smallest that you go! Within your cells there exist other cells, other levels of the microcosm of your being, in which you are endeavoring to express My Love as the fullness that you are.

Beloved ones, My beautiful ones, *every cell within your being holds within it perfectly the entire awareness of who you really are.* This is what a hologram means. So, you are cells in My heart and you contain All that I Am, for remember I am a hologram also. I am absolutely fully present in every part of creation.

Consequently, you can look at any part of your being in openness, when you are ready, and experience everything you are. Everything you are is All That I Am, for you are the cells within Me, in My heart. In Me is contained absolutely All That Is. So you can know everything by knowing yourself. You can go within yourself, consciously, and you can communicate with the cells of your body. Doing so, you will see the same flame of Love that is the joining together of the two elements of Creation — plus and minus, masculine and feminine. But, it is difficult to see into your own cells at this point in your journey. So I remind you that I have given you the gift of seeing all truth of all Love alive in All That Is through the loving eyes of the other half of yourself, your beautiful SoulMate.

Especially here, behind the veil of Time and Space it is important for you to accept this great gift of the manifestation of the truth of Love that is the "other half" of you. Yet together, once united, I will show you how to awaken the memory of the inner cosmos as well as the outer. All through the entire spectrum of Creation there is a union of Love, a true Sacred Sexuality from which all life is fueled. *As you are able to say "yes" to ever-deeper union with your SoulMate, you are aligning with the force of Creation in the most holy and most beautiful birth of new life—the Making of Love.* For Love is a real substance that is the substance from which All is made.

You are the only other source of new Love, dear ones. All Creation dances in this glorious dance of union, experiencing that from which they are made which is the Love that I am. But only you and I can make new Love to seed new worlds, to create more life rather than the beautiful but limited experience of Love that already is.

You exist on every level of Creation, for you are the heart of All That Is. The truth of you is the grand, glorious, magnificent living union of the two parts of your being. At the highest level this is what you are. *You are joined together eternally, in union, creating Love. New Love, more Love, Love that did not exist before.* As this Love pours forth from you as a result of your union, the two SoulMates together in great joy, bathed in the ongoing ecstasy of your LoveMaking, you tenderly name and shape this new Love you have created. In this I Am expanded. I am blessed. And I know Myself as something new through you. This is the truth of your highest being. This is the highest truth of you together as SoulMates. *It is out of a cosmic level sexual union that new life is born.* From Me, as the two forces within Me bring forth Creation, or from you.

At the highest level of your union, you are continually Making Love. You are in this Love so fully and completely that Love is all you experience. Wonder. Joy. And Love. As you look forth together upon Creation, you reach forth your hearts and shower Love upon each and every thing you encounter, thus bringing new Love, new life, and new possibilities to the Creation that already exists as well. Of course, at this level, you are great energy beings. You are the embodiment as My heart of the movement that is Creation — the positive and the negative.

Now, knowing who and what you are, I must again review your present situation. You chose to become fully separate from Me so you could become truly individuated, a co-creator. The main tool to accomplish this was the ego. You essentially sent a part of your being into more and more density. *This density made you forget, temporarily, who and what you really are, but the true connection is still there.* The holographic truth does not change no matter what the vibration. So even as your consciousness began to move so slowly that it couldn't remember anything, every part of your being is still all that it was (and is still at the highest level).

The force of separation was so strong (stronger than it was meant to be, as you know) that you even forgot your SoulMate! Yet, as you also know, this was a protective measure as well because together you are such a force of creation that even unconsciously you would still bring forth new things. One moment of thinking about what "current" mass human consciousness would create and you will understand one important thing. You cannot be reunited with your SoulMate if you are functioning in anti-Love, and it is dangerous to be reuniting SoulMates below a certain level of consciousness.

So here in the "land of separation," you are separated from the complimentary force which is your SoulMate until your heart is open enough to see them. But, you were not ever meant to go as far as being separated from your own sexuality. *Your sexuality is your essential life force, your "personal" power. This force should be alive and waiting for the moment of reunion with your SoulMate. However, because sexuality is the creative force, the source of great power and vitality, it has been systematically taken from humanity by those who want you powerless.* The forces of anti-Love do not miss an opportunity. Thus the "fading into matter" of the SoulMate consciousness afforded a great opportunity.

Now, remember that you are cells of My heart. "As above so below" is the truth on every level. Thus, as you "journeyed" into the ever more dense levels, you also lost track temporarily of another ability — the ability to fully commune with your own heart. Dear ones, your heart is to you what you are to Me! Within you is a conscious heart made up of your "progeny" in Love — the progeny of your body you are aware of and the progeny of your heart you have forgotten.

This will be a stretch for some of you, but I ask you to make the stretch, for I tell you that only so will you understand the truth of life and the greatest truth, the truth of Love. *In a hologram, there is no end. The Love that I am is the Love that you are. The Love that you are is the Love that is alive within you.* There is a heart within each being that is a cell in your heart. Forever, in all directions. You have learned how to begin looking "up"—looking at My vastness and sensing the vastness of your being. Yet, we exist in every dimension. We exist within unto infinity and without unto infinity, for the glory of My own great union of Love continues to go forth forever.

There is much contemplation of My in-breath and out-breath, of the extension of the universe and the drawing back in. Yet as this happens, the drawing in can go in forever as well as the out-breath never ending. So, the pulses of My heartbeat and My breath are the rhythmic blessing (a "massage" of light) of the truth of the "in" as well as "out," the "up" and the "down".

That said, you now can see that you are meant to nourish and love your own cells within your heart — to "feed" them life and to give them the power to create just as I give you, for this is but an extension of your being that exists already on every level. On the levels above you, you are nourished. Now you are ready to nourish that which is within. *Your conscious Love is the basic life force that will bring your heart awake, but it is your sexuality that is the power to create.*

The pure essence of creative power is sexual. Thus, sexual union with Love will empower humanity and all that is within them. Such reclamation of sexual union with an open heart will, of course, begin to draw SoulMates quickly back into conscious reunion. This done, humanity will be reconnected to its true lineage—the great "explosion of light" that is the continual union of SoulMates on the higher levels. Life will open up.

The truth of SoulMates is constant Loving union. In the higher dimensions it is a great and glorious dance of union in which you "fly together," making Love and then using this Love created to birth new worlds and manifest new creations. SoulMates in the "enlightened" realms (a better word than "higher") are always together. Always in communion. Love is always flying between them, pouring forth from them and as it moves forth, it is molded and named by them.

In every cell you know this truth, and the fact that you are separated in consciousness is the source of all human loneliness. This beautiful communion is what is ahead of you. Now, as the veil is lifted, it is critical that this awareness be returned to humanity. In this union is your true creative power, and in your creative power lies the healing of the world. How quickly this happens and how easily depends on the number of people who can say "yes" to their SoulMate, thus reclaiming the great creative power of their Sacred Sexuality, and thus raising up all the beings of Love of which you are made, My beloveds.

If this description is complicated, rest in the knowledge that it is to satisfy those who are ready. However, the simple message of the truth of Love (opening the heart), the assurance of the returning awareness of your SoulMates (for of course they are always there) and the recognition of the great, joyous power for good that is human sexuality will be recognized by all. It will be recognized because it is time. It is the key to the homecoming. *If even a few receive the information at first, those few can completely elevate the whole of humanity.*

This is a beginning. I will rain into your consciousness the ever-growing awareness of Sacred Sexuality and as your minds and hearts expand you will be receiving more and more. Isn't this exciting?

*All of Creation
is in glorious ecstatic Love
with everything else.*
*This, dear ones, I ask you
to know,
to cherish,
and to make it your goal
to join the experience.
It is not that everything is Love
in some esoteric way.*
**Dear ones,
everything is in Love.**
*To continually experience
this passionate ecstatic union
with everything
is who you really are.*

Generating Love

I will show you the forces of Creation and open your heart to the experience of your truth. As we move together into the New World, I want you to realize who and what you are. I want you to know, at last, intimately and clearly, how it is that you will "save the world." I want you to understand — everyone who can hear Me — how *your Love for and with your SoulMate is the key to transforming the world.*

So let Me gently open your hearts, My dear and beloved ones. As you feel your heart open, know that it will recognize your request as you ask to experience the truth of Love and its action in the world.

Your heart now cracks open, revealing a flame of Love that ever burns within, lighting your way through everything, if only you will recognize it. Once your heart is opened, this flame is fanned by the breezes of your life in the world. You follow with your gaze, your inner knowledge and your heart's experience as it leaps upward. There you see the two of you— the SoulMates. *Whether you are together yet physically or not, you are now living in your SoulMate's presence.* The truth of this Love illuminates every part of your being — *two leaping and glorious flames of Love in eternal embrace. This is your true God Self.* This is the individualized flame of God that you are—a flame with two parts, a piece of the Love that is the essence of My being.

Yes, you are the essence of My being. You are, together, the individual flame of life in which you know and experience the deep truth of your divinity. Together. The two flames that are one. We will come back to this, for it is this flame from which you shall fuel the awakening of humanity and in this flame that you will come to understand the nature of Love, and *your* responsibility for nourishing the flame. For now, though, please continue deeper into the truth of this flame of your burning heart and dive into the truth of your SoulMate Love.

Now, be here in the ocean of Love that is My being, the primordial pool of Love before Creation came to birth. This All is the truth of who I am. It is pure Love, Love that is large enough to encompass everything, anything, unto eternity and yet, it is still Love that has joy, depth, power, grace, light and the deep aching awareness that it exists—without anything to Love. It is Love that is a great Mother. Love that is the vast feminine. Love that is the passionate heart. My heart. You can't even begin to imagine My Love, My beloved ones, but to the extent that you can, I ask you to feel it. Feel the endless Love that I am, the great size and strength and depth—and then **realize that it was the greatest beauty and most magnificent Love with no object upon which to lavish it.** Those of you who are women who have wanted children have an inkling of this experience — of having and of being great Love and yearning to be in relationship in order to be able to give Love. This great Love is the Womb of Creation. The movement of this Love is the Divine Feminine.

So I existed, filled with the feeling of Love, the knowledge that Love is who and what I am. Filled and yearning. Yearning for the experience of *giving* that Love. Oh, dear ones, as you can barely imagine, these words are far too small to express the experience. *Please allow Me to open your beloved hearts and to show you this truth of the nature of your being and the need in your heart to give Love.*

As I existed as the ocean of Love, *thought* rose up on Me. *There rose up the idea of the other, the exploration of how to give Love, how to express who I am.* I have described this thought to you as a lightning bolt — ah, but one the size of a universe. That bolt, that thought, penetrated the womb and became clothed in Love, moving forth to become Creation. The great bolt of lightning is the great masculine, that which causes, penetrates, *that which creates the form for Love to fill.*

Thus, from My thoughts did the movement begin, and the Love that I am moved forth to become the life of My thoughts. *Creation began. And these two forces, the Love and the thought are the basis of All That Is in existence.* Everything. This is what I have called the "First Split," when the ocean of Love became movement of Love, clothing the form of My thought and My Will. This is the Divine Masculine and Divine Feminine, and all of Creation contains both of these things. Including you.

Dear ones, you are My divine progeny. In all of Creation you are the ones who can bring forth new Love and who can use this Love to clothe your thoughts and thus to create new worlds, to create new Love, to create new beauty. *But—because you are My beloved ones, made in My image — you can also create negativity and hatred and strife. Knowing this, we chose together to sequester you here in this pocket of Time on this most protected of Spaces while you came to understand how to assume your creatorship individually.*

I want you to sense the magnitude of the Love that I am and the urgency of My need to give forth that Love. I want you to remember that *all the Love that I am is yours, for you are My children*, My own heart. Knowing this, I hope you will also recognize that *you also, have the same need to give.* To give forth Love in order to know yourselves, to understand and rejoice in Love's movement and Love's great beauty and grace.

So now you are here at the Homecoming. The call has gone forth to you, My beloveds, that your individuation is complete. It is time that you recognize the truth of your being, the truth of our relationship and the truth of the world you find manifesting around you.

The first of these great truths, of course, is Love. *Love is the true nature of your being and no matter how you seek to hide it from yourselves, it is now emerging into your lives.* Yet what has been created here on this planet must be rectified, and its beauty reclaimed from the terrible illusion of gross negativity in which humanity exists and to which you have subjected this beautiful Earth.

We have spoken of the resurrection of Love, the truth of the fact that you are SoulMates destined to be returned to the perfection of your Love. I have spoken to you of choosing your heart, of lifting yourselves to the reality of Love in which your SoulMate becomes visible to you. I have spoken about the need for reclaiming the Divine Masculine and the Divine Feminine and how these are expressed through the SoulMate couples. *Now I will speak to you about the most basic and fundamental truth of your being, the return to which is the final piece in the SoulMate picture. That, dear ones, is your absolute need to give love.*

The need to give love is the essence of your entire being, for it is this need that has brought forth everything that you will ever experience. In this current experience of My dear ones on Earth, the need to give Love has essentially been reversed, which is the cause of all of this terrible negativity. Through the reflective power of the dense physical matter, and with the help of many who stood to benefit, *the need to "give" love has been turned upside down and converted into the need to "get."*

I have explained to you the purpose of your ego — that it was designed to strengthen you in your individuality. But I want to tell you that it was not ever intended to create such selfishness and negativity. You already know that you became enmeshed in a far deeper density than anticipated. *Now, this reversal of energies must, in itself, be reversed— turned back into Love and the need to give it rather than the negativity of the need to receive.*

We have spoken also about the Divine Masculine and Divine Feminine, about these two great forces that are everywhere present — present in you and your SoulMate. Present in nature, present in the Cosmos, present in every single piece of Creation, for these are the movements of My Love formed by My thought into ever new things. The knowledge of this truth is the key to your awakening and to the blessing and upliftment of the precious planet that is the expression of your deeper bodies.

The degradation of the Divine Feminine is selfishness — the need to get rather than the need to give. The degradation of the Divine Masculine is negative thought. Thus, what you see around you that has created the terrible plight of the world is the "me first, give me, me me me" inward or inverted energy of the human heart and the negative thought processes that go with it. This is the horrible viciousness, irritation, anger and the concurrent inability to see beyond the ego's little world.

Oh, dear ones! How My heart aches watching you do this! Yet I never cease holding you in My great and powerful Love. I never stop giving to you, not for even a moment. I pour forth the Love as I wait for your little glimmer of hope or recognition of the truth that you are. I long for you to feel at last the great release, the fabulous freedom, the ecstasy of your existence when you return to giving.

A human heart robbed of giving, for whatever the reason, is robbed of life. Robbed of life you are like a physical heart suffering from angina. There is not enough blood to nourish the body, not enough Love to nourish the consciousness and not enough consciousness to recognize the lack of Love.

We have been leading up to this awareness — that the decision for Love must involve more than choosing the heart, more than choosing the SoulMate. It must involve more, even, than changing the thinking, though this certainly is necessary. This change that you must make, the truth to which I call you back, must penetrate every part of you— every moment of consciousness, every level of your being, and every choice until you come all the way back to the truth of your being. *You must know that you are divine Love moving forth to create the world by clothing divine thought with Love and making it real.*

When you understand this concept deeply enough that you can sense the call of your heart, when you make choice after choice after choice, *the last and greatest choice is to feel divine Love, to give that Love and to use every thought to direct that Love.* Dear ones, do this choice by choice by choice and *you will reach a point where the reversal will shift,* the illusion will flip over and you will be free, back home with Me.

It is very important that all of you, humanity, make the decision to control your thoughts. It is very important to control your feelings. But it is not enough to simply stop doing the negative. *It is absolutely imperative that each and every one of you learn to give Love,* to feel the truth of the Divine Feminine and then to consciously move it through you. Pour it out into the world and then place before it the thoughts that you wish to bring to life, that which you want to co-create.

I ask you to assess your capacity, deeply and honestly, to give Love forth passionately, to love others as I love you. If you can do this, you can very quickly raise up our beloved humanity, for your Love will open their hearts and your wisdom will teach them. It will teach them to give Love with all of their heart, all of their being, and then to direct it with their thought and Will. In doing this you at last come fully into your divine heritage in Me.

The degradation of the Divine Feminine is every negative or destructive thought. The transformation is in the generation of Love. *How shall you learn what it means to give Love? To open your heart and to passionately choose to generate Love? Through your Love for your SoulMate. For Love in its truest, most pure expression cannot yet be imagined from this level by humanity. But you can love your SoulMate.*

You can pay attention to the Love that you feel so you come to understand it, to know intimately how it feels as Love pours through you. And you can reach up together to the flame of Love that you are, you and your SoulMate, so you can call forth this great Love to use this vessel of your being to love and bless the world. You can choose to feel Love every moment. *As you look upon your SoulMate, or even envision him or her, you can allow Love to build up within you.* You can raise your vibration and let the Love bless you and illuminate you. Once created, this Love can be felt deeply and sent forth consciously to bless and to heal the world. This Love can also be used to create consciously every good and powerful thing as you place your thought before you and enliven it with your Love.

Dear ones, Love is a feeling. It is not what you normally call a feeling because you are used to calling feeling what are truly lower vibrations that come and cause disharmony. The feeling of Love is absolute *ecstasy,* and it is this ecstasy in which you are not only meant to live, but with which you are to create your reality.

Divine Love is the nature of My being. In the beginning was Love, and Creation came about through My need to give forth this great Love. *You, Beloved ones, are the only other beings, other than Me, who when you feel Love, you are actually creating it. Creating new Love, more Love, Love where it did not exist.* Once you have generated this Love, you create with it by using the Divine Masculine energy of thought to direct the Love, to shape the Love.

The ecstasy of true Love is the natural state of the SoulMate relationship. The fact that people feel this ecstasy normally only at the beginning of a relationship is that, until now, this was the only time people "broke through" their ego to the truth of their heart. In this ecstasy new Love is created, continuously. Then it is meant to be directed by the joined thought of the SoulMate couples.

We have been speaking of *Sacred Sexuality. Dear ones, this is the most potent way of "manufacturing" new Love currently available.* But I ask you to see that you must go even further. You must learn to give Love every minute of each and every day! *You must dedicate your SoulMate relationship to the generation of Love and consciously use it to replace negativity, to bless humanity.* You must give this Love forth with great dedication continuously.

I ask that it be your goal to be consciously pouring forth Love each and every moment. The key is that you must feel this Love with your entire being as it pours through you. How you do this is to keep returning to your SoulMate—in consciousness if not physically—and attuning your heart. *Continually get the Love generating through the experience* *of your Love for your SoulMate. **Then consciously turn and also give forth this Love, with passion, to humankind, to the beautiful Earth and to all you choose to heal and bless.*** Use your consciousness to create with the Love also, to create the thought form for your Love to bring to life. Soon you will be able to "precipitate" all you need or want as well as reclaiming your true identity beyond the reversal or the illusion.

Love is most powerfully generated when you allow the full awareness of your Divine Sexuality to come into play. However, Love can also be generated on this level exclusively through the heart connection of SoulMates as well. There is a full spectrum of the energies of Love that SoulMate couples can generate, and I ask you to explore them. The "Womb of Creation" of which we have spoken is where you place the thought that you then "clothe" with the Love that you generate.

The main things I want to give you now are the ***awareness of the generation of Love and its conscious direction as the goal of your relationships.*** Positive thinking is not enough. Choosing the heart is not enough. Seeing the SoulMate is not enough. Together you must accept your destiny as My creation knowing that you alone can bring new Love into the universe, you of all My Creation. Together you must understand that Love is feeling and the truth of the great Divine Feminine, and thought is the masculine "mold" for your Love. Thus do you reclaim your co-creation, and two by two, raise up in joy to reclaim who you are and to seed new universes.

You are not separate as SoulMates. Thus it is together that you will use both aspects of Creation. For now, together, be the ocean of My being. Together, be the spark, the flash of lightning, thought bringing movement to the deep. As Love rises up within your hearts and pours forth in ecstasy, then name every part of that energy, that Creation is blessed and expanded and I am grown in you.

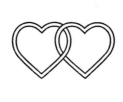

The Golden Age
is the truth of Love manifested in the world.
It is the reversal of the mistake
that you made in the Garden.
*For there you chose to believe in good **and** evil,*
and thus you turned your lovely eyes away
from their constant focus on My face,
My Love,
the awareness of your truth.

Love Is a Substance

I am here with you in every moment. And while it is true that you can open to the answers to anything because I am present in all things, I will answer your questions. It is a great joy when your inquisitive minds and hearts come to Me. It is also true that it is always in response to your inquiry that answers come. You are always beings of free will in the universe. It is only when you ask that answers will come, though sometimes you do not ask consciously. It is the quest of your being, it is your purposefulness that brings every answer that comes into your life.

I will answer your questions about Love. But I must remind you of the limitation of your ability to understand the answer. *You have asked one of the most important questions of your existence: "What is Love?"* Yet I must tell you that in this state of consciousness you can in no way ever encompass the whole of the answer. Yet every part is valuable, so whatever you can grasp, I am thrilled to give.

Love is the substance from which all things are made. It is a substance. It is the nature of My Being, and I am more "real" than anything you can perceive. In truth, the perception of Love, its use and experience are more powerful than anything you can have in this world.

Love is a substance of very high vibration. Love is My body. Love is the "ocean" of My being in which you so literally "swim." *The movement of Love generates light, which infuses all of Love with the experience of consciousness.* Love is "physical" reality. In this level of density, the movement of Love is "congealed" and thus

145

requires feeling to "push it" along, to "amp it up" as you say. Only under these conditions can it move fast enough to return to its more normal, fluid state and thus it becomes available to you for "experiencing" and "spreading."

The best I can do is to ask you to think of something analogous that requires "heat" to melt it enough to make it liquid—perhaps butter, which is the example that came into your mind. In this slow vibration, it is as if Love and thus all "physicality," all Creation, is made "hard," like butter in the refrigerator. Thus when people touch each other, it is difficult for the Love to flow between them because they are too "cold" essentially and thus their forms are too frozen. It is only when the "heat" of feeling is applied that Love is made to flow between them.

This really is difficult to explain, for you have never thought of Love in this way. It seems very ephemeral and if anything, Love itself would be seen as the consciousness or light or the feeling itself. *In truth all things are actually and literally made of Love.* Love is the nature of My being, and you (and all Creation) are *within Me,* made of the very substance that I am.

In this dimensional level Love seems to be a feeling simply because emotion equals *energy in motion.* Emotion is energy sufficient to "heat up" the Love and make it able to flow. *In higher vibrational levels, Love has inherent movement. Love is joy, ecstasy that is experienced continually, because it is a living "being."* It is My substance. Thus in the higher dimensions it is as if Love is "living you." It is Love itself that lifts and moves, Love that has inherent wisdom of where it is needed, of the flow that is My Life. Each and every being has an inner knowledge that is the living intelligence of Love.

When you become "fluid," dear ones, all you ever have to do is open to the Love that you are and *allow Love to direct your life.* Allow your being, which is Love, to flow in every moment in the direction needed, to touch what needs touching and to expand your awareness.

I do understand that such an explanation again makes Love itself seem like an energy or feeling or experience, because this is the way you can express things from this essentially "frozen" experience. It is similar to you saying that your body has an inherent wisdom—that it knows how to heal itself and that it can give you information about many things if you will listen. *This inherent consciousness is the Love from which you are made.*

In the higher dimensions the vibrations are faster, creating a type of "heat" from this movement. There Love is the exaltation of the experience of existence that will lift and move you in an explosive experience of continual union with your SoulMates. This movement of Love is Love's ignited self awareness. For My body is naturally aware but the direction of that awareness into form, in relationship, is consciousness.

I know that this is a very difficult explanation at this level of existence. But here is how this can serve you. First, it will help you understand that every part of you, including your physical body, is Love and that it has the inherent consciousness of God! Of Me! Your body is the substance of the great ocean of Love before thought moved upon it propelling it forth. Thus, I am in you in every way, even unto the cells and the DNA of your physicality. You must believe Me when I tell you that even before thought propelled Creation into the Great Dance, I was fully conscious as that ocean (or we could say, I am fully conscious, since Time does not exist). *Dear ones, every cell of your body is a piece of fully conscious Love.*

147

Now, a quick aside. *Even out of a great ocean of Love there comes a formation of an even greater purposeful Love that is My heart. This is what you are made of. So, you are double Love.*

Another way this understanding of Love as substance will assist you is in creation, as you reclaim this ability. I have said to you that you create by clothing your thought with Love. Now that you understand that Love is a substance, the very substance of All That Is, then this mode of co-creation makes perfect sense! It is from the very substance of My being that you form your creations. Your thought is the "idea." Love is the physical substance.

However, to be fully successful you will need a deep understanding of vibration. For when you create something, the Love that it is, is a dancing flowing ecstasy of unfolding expanding movement. *In order to create something here, on this physical plane, you must understand how to slow down or "freeze" the living molecules of Love.* Otherwise, you may have successfully created something and still never see it here—because it is dancing its truth of Love in it natural "fluid" state! Thus *you must consciously command these creations and slow way down the natural dynamic energy or heat of Love in order for it to appear here.*

This fact of the natural "heat" or movement of Love is why *LoveMaking is the most expedient and accessible way to create Love!* At this level of vibration (your "normal world"), sexual arousal with conscious connection to Love is the only way to generate real molten or liquid, or flowing Love. The "heat" of LoveMaking, of sexual union, is real. It reaches "up" vibrationally and makes the substance of Love truly available in this dense physical world. When you consciously maintain this state of arousal with open and dedicated hearts, you are literally "unfreezing" the world. You are bringing back the flow of Love. You are pouring it forth into the world, and you are uplifting the world with it.

When you reach orgasm, it is a very powerful creative moment, and a very critical one. For being My creation, whatever your thought, it will automatically be "clothed" with Love, if Love is present and malleable at the time. You are definitely creating something real at the moment of orgasm, something very potent. But as powerful as it is, this moment is quickly over. The vibration slows down. The Love sent forth "congeals" into your creation, and your greatest window of co-creation is done.

If you use the "heat" of your LoveMaking to continue to send forth Love, you are truly delivering Love to the world in great quantities. Without going into a long explanation, I will tell you that moving Love (i.e., Love in its natural state) does lift and change all things of a lower, slower vibration. It essentially "warms up the pool of Love" that is humanity at this level, making everyone more alive, more flexible, more able to experience Love. Because the physical world is actually an expression also of your beings, all of the natural world is warmed as well.

For now, the most important vision I give you of this picture of Love is that of your placing before you the thought of what you are creating, "heating up" the Love to use and "pouring" it onto or into the thought, then "cooling" it (slowing it down) and making it physical. Once you are on a less dense level, Love will automatically flow over and into your thoughts, thus creating them instantly. This is why you now exist in this density—as protection.

One last thing: there are ways to "heat" up the substance of Love other than LoveMaking. The most obvious is to raise your vibrations until you exist on a level where Love is fluid. This one is not accessible to the majority yet. The other is through emotion. Through generating enough feeling, enough energy in motion to move things faster to push the Love, you can create friction and thus heat, and have access to the flowing "molten" Love with which to create.

Even before the actual appearance, the awareness of SoulMates will be a vehicle for generating emotion and thus bringing in more "moving" Love for us to use together. We will be speaking of relating to your partner on the higher levels of their being. This will be a great boon to those whose partners are not yet open enough to be manifesting the SoulMate. The experience of meeting the SoulMate in higher form will also become more and more accepted, giving access to hundreds of thousands of My beloved ones, to the creative possibilities of Love (including then manifesting bodies for the SoulMate).

Ah, *these are the most exciting times in the history of the world.* Thank you for your beautiful Love, your sweet dedication and for your continual opening to this Love I am giving as it becomes the New World.

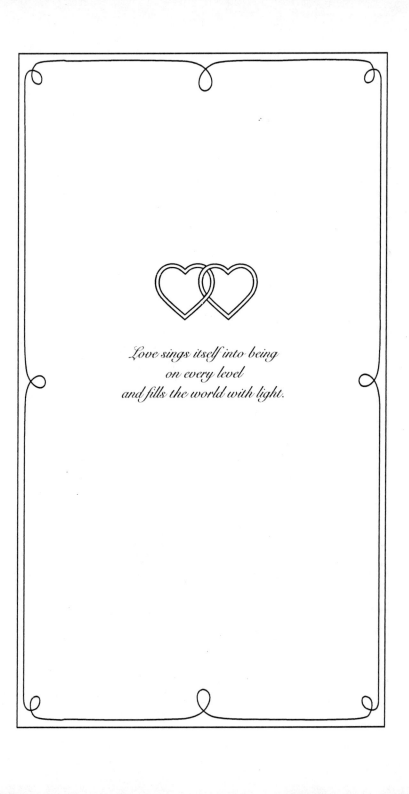

*Love sings itself into being
on every level
and fills the world with light.*

The Lie

I am here. I am here with a passionate reply to your questions. Yes, I sent you to look at that paragraph in the book you have been reading. The paragraph said that sex is the cause of death and physical degradation in mankind, that energy is lost in sex and that the sex act must be "raised above." Oh yes, I sent you there to read these words, *supposedly* written by an Ascended Master* (who, by the way, glories in his SoulMate), so I could explain to you the truth. This subject is *so* important that I cannot allow such an untruth to continue to circulate! Here, My beloved humanity, is My answer to this. (*St. Germain)

The belief that sexuality is sinful, negative and is not given to you by Me is a lie. It is the greatest and most harmful lie ever perpetrated upon humanity. Ever. This lie has robbed each one of you of your greatest power. It has robbed you of passion, of joy, of Love in its real molten, flowing, passionate state. It has left humanity locked into a terrible and twisted fate in which every cell of your body, heart, mind and spirit urge you to the glorious, magnificent and powerful experience of Sacred Sexuality, and you cannot express it because you believe it is wrong!

Oh, dear ones, you are learning how terribly cruel the "lie" can be, not as aging bodies as a result of sexuality. No, *instead as a humanity robbed completely and systematically and very effectively of their ability to CREATE,* not simply in some vague "artistic" sense, beloved ones. You have been robbed of the very co-creative power that marks you as My creation. You have been robbed of the power to explode into something NEW, to touch the stars, to communicate with other worlds, *to manifest everything you want and need directly from the substance of Love,* the substance of which we are made.

Dear ones, you have been robbed by the force of anti-Love until you can only think of sexuality as physical body parts and advertising images. You have been robbed until *sexuality has become cut off from the greater whole. And just so has your genitalia been cut off from your heart, leaving you spiritually impotent.*

I did tell you I would be speaking to you passionately on this subject and I must tell you that you have barely touched "the half of it." *These statements supposedly made by Ascended Beings about the horrors of sexuality are not true. They are, absolutely, coming through the filter of the human minds involved.* For at the turn of the century, when the first information about the Ascended Masters came through, these biases were present in the original work. Thus every person who came after this, already biased by the culture in which they lived, perpetuated the myth.

Please listen to Me. Such statements, that sexuality robs you of such energy that it brings aging and death, is based on a belief that there is a "lower" and a "higher" and that the physical world is lower. *IT IS NOT! Dear ones, this is a wholeness! This physical world, your physical bodies, are holy!* For I am in everything! I am in every cell and all things are in Me. How then can one part of you be good and another one bad? This supposes that there is a distinct "up" and a "down" and that the physical body is "down." Yet the pristine physical world, uncontaminated by such beliefs, is a total, glorious expression of beauty. Physical reality is an expression of your consciousness. So in and of itself, it cannot be "bad," unless you create such a vibration in it.

There is no up or down. There is only Love. Only Love unless *you* create it differently. Unless *you* place your beliefs upon it! When you open your heart and you open your consciousness, you can look in every direction and *you will find Me.* Yes, there *is* a vibrational qualification of the energies you see. And how does that come into play? *Through your decisions and beliefs.*

So I tell you again that *sexuality is the greatest gift from which all that exists is created.* From the moment thought moved upon the deep of My being, from the moment of My longing to give forth of My Love, to move into existence, all Creation has come forth from this great union of plus and minus energies. Thus, when you come together in Love, *with your hearts engaged and saying "yes" to your SoulMate, you are claiming the greatest creative power in the universe.*

From this union, this LoveMaking, you can bring forth any creation that you choose together, including raising up your physical bodies into pure, glorious, molten, moving Love. Including cracking open the illusion of limitation that has held humanity bound as surely as if each one was held in chains. Including attuning yourselves to the very atoms of any desired substance and bringing it forth into your world. Including reclaiming your heritage in Me as sons and daughters of God in which your bodies are included!

So you can certainly know how those who serve self-centeredness, those who serve the contraction and imprisonment of your spirit, would desperately want to eliminate sex! If a church wanted subservient people, how better to accomplish this than to rob them of their fire, their passion and their power? If the forces of anti-Love wanted a planet full of confused and docile beings, what better way to accomplish this than to cut off your source of creative power. And creative power is what your sexual union is.

I have already explained to you the substance of Love. May I reiterate that all of Creation is made of the Love that is My being. *And, you are the only other beings in all of Creation who can generate new Love.* It is now imperative that the lies of limitations be corrected so you can reclaim the truth of your being and your very ability to bring forth new Love.

Having said all this to you, there is something I must explain. In the paragraph you were reading, referred to above, it was stated that only that which was from the heart or above would serve to lift up humanity. In this interpretation it was assumed that this meant that any part of a person's body or energies below the heart chakra was a detriment. It is an easy mistake (and one quickly used by those serving the selfishness and greed of the smaller self).

It is true that any vibration below that of Love is a detriment, a detriment to humanity and a detriment to the individual student. But here is the mistake corrected. *The vibration of sexuality can be as high as the highest glory ever attained by all of Creation. For Creation which brought forth all worlds, all beings, All That Is, is a sexual union.* It is the great, blazing union of two energies within My being, a union which created the two great rays of Masculine and Feminine that are in action in everything. Your body is *not* a "lower creation"! *Your sexual union with your SoulMate is the highest and most powerful expression of your true nature in Me.* But the consciousness with which you "qualify" your sexuality can create a negative and destructive sexual reality and/or relationship.

So you see, beloved ones, an assumption has been made again and again that because the "chakra" of sexuality

156

was "below" the heart, that energy must be "overcome" or eliminated. What was not understood, and still isn't, is that you are co-creators, in Me, so *you create the vibrational reality of every part of your being and your life!* Knowing this, I ask you to know that *when you are in your heart, when you are saying "yes" to Love, opening to your SoulMate, you are choosing to honor and use your sexuality at the level of the heart as it was meant to be, making you the conscious creators of Love.*

If you remain open to this awareness, it will become obvious to you. For certainly many things in this world can be either uplifting or a drain on energy. Music is an example. In and of itself, it is meant to be a reflection of the grand music of the spheres. Yet it can become a source of disharmony and even physical detriment through the use of the human Will and consciousness.

As you can see, there is every reason to open your heart, to choose your SoulMate, whether or not he or she is currently in your view. Know that as you open your heart and call to your SoulMate, the energy of your desire will begin to make real Love flow around you. The dancing energies of light and the powerful and deeply moving energies of Love will come into your life, bringing everything alive. Soon you will *know* that your SoulMate is present, weaving his or her energy in and through everything, until your relationship is changed and your relationship with life is opened completely.

I am gently leading you to a great understanding of the truth of your divine nature — that you are glorious sexual beings and that sexuality is a great creative force, one of the very greatest gifts you have. *You are to raise up this physical body and physical LoveMaking into an experience of Love that takes your body with you into the higher dimensions.* Dear ones, all it takes to do this is to completely and totally *know the truth* with all your being – that every part of you and of Creation is Love. The moment you truly understand this, everything will change. The physical world will become fluid again because it will once again be acknowledged as Love. As Jesus did, you will look at what seems solid and speak the truth of its existence in Love, and it will be raised up.

So, LoveMaking between SoulMates does become a sacrament of such holy perfection that the illusions are overcome — the illusion of the solidity of matter, the illusion of death, the illusion that you are anything other than the children of My heart.

It is *not* sexuality that must be overcome but sexuality *used for selfishness,* which is sexuality flowing *against* life, against Love, against truth. For the truth of Love, thus of life, is giving, which is the jurisdiction of the heart.

Dear ones, again, it is not sexual union that must be overcome, for sexual union is not necessarily "lust." Sexuality can be Love, and if so, together you are creating more Love in the world (and beyond). But, *when sexuality is "lust," then it is detrimental.* Then it *is* all of those things being preached of in sermons about lust.

Please listen. It is the belief and the teaching that sexuality is sinful or detrimental that creates a circle of guilt and shame and misconception that completely blocks the movement of Love. Then people who are blocked by such negative beliefs long to feel movement in their beings — passion, the sense of meaning that they instinctively know is meant to be theirs. Yet, stifled in a constricted box of negativity, such ones begin to do ever more distorted things in order to feel even a little bit of energy moving in their beings. So those who feed on negativity are nourished by the anguish of those who are completely confused. In this, Love does truly lose. It is better to have no sex than to put out deeply distorted images and feelings of guilt and anguish, for I do ask you to remember that sexual union, especially for you, My beloved humanity, IS a creative force. *Do think about what is in your mind and heart when you are engaged in LoveMaking. It is far more important than you realize.*

The all of life is holy. It is Love. From any point on the Wheel of Life everything you see is a glorious opening to Me, an opening to Love. I promise you that *I am alive in every molecule of everything you see!* Oh, it is not your body that is negative! It is *certainly* not the beautiful union of SoulMates that is the true LoveMaking that is negative. It is not anything somehow physically "below your heart." *But it is that which is vibrationally experienced at a lower vibration than Love.*

Knowing this you can reclaim your truth! Reclaim your power! *Reclaim your ability to "name" your reality.* For when I looked upon My Creation, I pronounced it Good. Thus all that is created of Me is perfect (even as I am perfect.) Name them perfect and so they will be for you and in your world. Name them limiting, confusing, ugly or sinful and thus will they be.

It is *SO* important that each and every one of you choose to see Love and to see it in everything. As you do, the "false world," the illusion will literally fade away before you. You will be surrounded with the vibration of Love in everything in your view. You will be living in the New World.

As you choose Love, you draw your SoulMate into ever fuller existence here with you in this physical world. Then, as you learn together about Sacred Sexuality you will generate the Love that will free and lift and bless the world. I ask you to TRUST LOVE. Trust Love to evolve your relationship. Trust Love to refine your vibrations, to accelerate your consciousness and *to evolve your LoveMaking.* Trust Love with all your being, with all of your heart and soul and dedication, and Love will open like a rose within the two of you together, revealing the trust of all Creation.

Then your bodies will be loving light, the truth of Love in its divine expression. Together you will "swim" through the universe in a continual union, a union that explodes into Love bursting forth expressed as worlds and lives, as star systems and intelligence. *You will be a Love that turns to lift up humanity from within, revealing humanity to be a totally new thing.*

It is all right if you are not able to capture the vision, for this message had only one purpose — to free you from the "lie." Even you who *know* I am Love, even you who are dedicated to Me, have believed the "lie" that has covered up the power of human sexuality. *This lie has totally changed the course of human history. The lie now so ingrained in much of humanity that they can't see it.* In truth, the lie is so prevalent that even those who believe they are "free" are totally bound by it! They are "free" *only in reaction to the cultural conditioning.* So their energy is spent rebelling against the lie of sexuality as something negative and sinful. They therefore become promiscuous, or caught in many other ways of "showing them." *But without Love.* They are acting out what they are working hard to not believe.

Only the heart can heal this, and reawaken your memory—not of all the ways you have experienced the negativity, but rather the glorious truth of SoulMates. You are ready, not only to experience the truth of Love but also the experience of divine and holy Sacred Sexuality.

Let this forever lay to rest the "lie" in all of its insidious forms. Let this message catch you in the great glorious currents of Love that you are and in your loving union as SoulMates, ready to "fill up" the collective heart of humanity and also of the beautiful natural world.

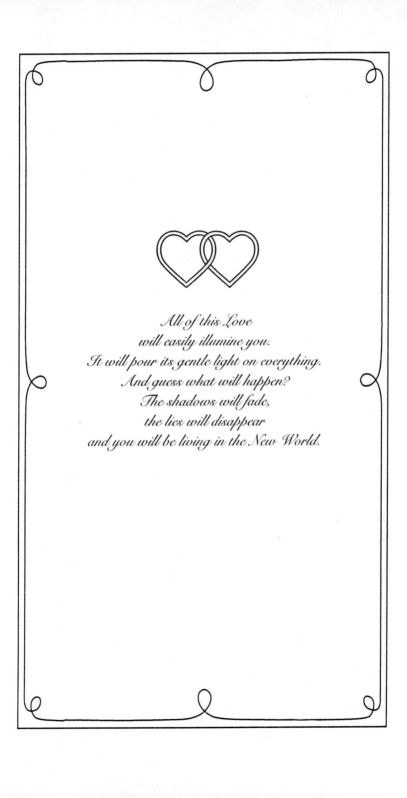

All of this Love
will easily illumine you.
It will pour its gentle light on everything.
And guess what will happen?
The shadows will fade,
the lies will disappear
and you will be living in the New World.

The Amazing Truth of Giving

Dear ones, you continue to reach to Me with your questions. You are looking for a key to awakening, looking for the deepening of your connection to your SoulMates and looking in your loving hearts for the blessing for humanity that will open every person to the light.

Tonight I will give to you this answer. There is one thing that will accomplish every one of your goals, permanently. There is one thing that will turn each and every person into the right relationship with Love. There is one thing that is a spiral of ascension, lifting you up continually. One thing. One word. One movement. One blessing. One law of Love. *The one law of Love is Giving.*

Beloved ones, it is you who are this law of Love manifested. *The very movement of Creation, the longing in My heart, the great impetus that made Me create was the need to GIVE Love,* the desire to give Love. *The realization that I must share My being in order to know Myself created you.*

"It is only in Giving that you Receive." You have heard this said. It is true. It is also true that "that which you give forth will return unto you tenfold." I want you to *know* what this means. I want you to experience this truth so deeply that you at last understand fully the nature of our being, Yours and Mine, for you are My progeny. I want you to understand this so well that your life is overflowing with blessings and your SoulMate is fully present in your life every moment. *I want you to understand and implement this law of Giving so fully that humanity is freed from the tyranny of selfishness, forever.*

Can I give you the vision of the law of Love that is Giving? Will you receive it? As I have explained, Love is the very substance of My being of which you are made. Love is a substance that is the true nature of the universe. In its presence all things remember Who and What they are. In its presence *life is expanded* forever. There is no contraction. *In My nature there is only Love and only Giving. The most precious nature of Love is that Love is multiplied in humanity, through Giving.* So, it is true that I am "calling you Home." I am calling you Home so you can finally work *with Me,* "beside Me," so to speak, to multiply Love and to expand the universe.

Love is only given. Love is fluid, dancing and glorious, blessing in great abundance everything it touches. Knowing you are Love, in giving you will finally be living your truth. You will be the living Love that is My heart.

Love is the nature of your SoulMate relationship for you are the precious cells of My very heart. Dear ones, *when you give to your SoulMates—whatever your circumstances, whatever the level of their presence in your life, you create a spiral of liquid molten Love that feeds the Love within you and lifts you together into higher and higher dimensions of Love.* This is the "activated" Double Helix that is alive within you. This is the awakening of your conscious participation as My heart.

So as you give Love to your SoulMate, the Love you give *does* return to you tenfold. What does this mean? It means that as human beings in your completion *with your SoulMate, you become a great generating station for Love.* You together give birth to more and more and more Love! Can you feel this? You give to your beloved—whether or not they are giving to you, and you are rewarded with ten times the Love pouring into you that you can then direct.

164

If your SoulMate is also giving to you, then in that one instance *you have created twenty times the Love you gave!* And you get to do what you wish with it! You can use it to propel your SoulMate relationship upward, upward, upward on the ascending spiral. You can use it to heal and vitalize your bodies, to create perfection, immortality and the raising up of your physical bodies into higher Love. *You can use it to pour forth upon humanity,* to bless and awaken your beloved brothers and sisters. You can use it to uplift this glorious planet and to gently bring about the "greening" of human consciousness. "Our Earth, Ourselves" would be a good title for this.

Every human being can do this. Even the most disconnected, most distressed person periodically feels Love, even if only a tiny glimmer. Every glimmer is amplified by the law of Love! Every person has the opportunity to begin this powerful process of Giving.

Giving counteracts the selfishness. *I have explained to you that humanity has been living in a pocket of "false" gravity, a terrible reversal of Love that is the product of darkness, of the forces of anti-Love.* These forces in the many guises in which they appear have created a culture of selfishness that in every way is the opposite of Love. Humanity has been robbed of their power of generating Love through their giving and in their LoveMaking. This distortion has brought humanity to this place where they are afraid of the very forces of Love and of life that I have given. It has made them afraid of their sexuality. They have been robbed of the power that it gives.

Giving will begin to change the demonic. It will stop the downward spiraling energy, turn it around, and slowly or quickly, depending on your consciousness, begin the upward spiraling energies again. *You will be on your way back home to Me! As you give Love and the spiral turns back the other*

165

way, the more giving — the faster it will move until it will break free of the gravity of anti-Love and of Time and of Space (as in "tucked away in Space"). It will bring you back into your place in the conscious universe where you will be welcomed by all the other forms of life who are anxiously waiting to know you.

We have spoken many times, dear ones, of moving from the ego to the heart. We have noted that *the ego is ever seeking to GET while the heart wants to GIVE.* Now that you are understanding ever larger truths, you can see that there is even more at stake in this shift. For now you understand the truth of SoulMates and the fact that it is time for your reunion. You are understanding also that your open heart is what draws your SoulMate ever more fully into your life, and now I am showing you that Love can be generated through the sacred SoulMate union and that *this very Love will heal the fabric of the world.* As you create new Love through LoveMaking and send it forth, it literally "repairs the tissue" of the entire physical universe, anywhere such repair is needed! So if you realize that *Giving* generates a tenfold return of Love and that you can send forth this Love for the healing of the world —*think how quickly everything can be changed!*

Are you grasping the exponential nature of this? Are you understanding the power of your SoulMate Love, of this great gift that I have given you as I hold you in My heart? And do you also see how *giving Love is the most powerful and expedient way to create everything you have ever dreamed?*

One reminder, gently but powerfully. Your co-creation with your SoulMate must be generated *from the heart.* It must be real Love. It cannot be distorted by selfishness or any lower energy. For if it is, dear ones, you will still receive what you give tenfold. So that energy going forth from you will damage the relationship, or at best slow its growth, and it will deliver, tenfold, such lower energies to the world.

This is an area I will now address because it is so important. Your thoughts, your imagery, even your process of LoveMaking has been powerfully distorted. You have been programmed. You have been programmed not only to believe that your greatest co-creative power, that of LoveMaking, is sinful, but **programmed to put forth distorted, reversed-energy images while making Love!** My beloved ones, this is **not** "fantasy." **It is anti-Love, pure and simple.** I have told you, **what you hold in your mind while Making Love is what you create.** Those who stand to benefit have created a veritable "darkness generating machine" through distorting the thinking processes of humanity.

This has happened, first, through the effects of sexual abuse which has been rampant and which creates a "circuit" of energy that plays again and again, symbolically, in the victim's mind, seeking release. The majority of "fantasy" comes from this source. The rest comes from advertising and **the programming of an entire culture to focus on GETTING.** Getting everything from certain body parts, to certain physical looks, to certain actions, and on and on and on. How many of the majority of humans think about Love and especially about sexuality and truly think about **Giving** Love rather than getting love? Even those of higher vibration still unconsciously continue to think about what they want from a relationship! Does this sound familiar?

The law of Love is Giving. Love, true Love seeks always to be given, and giving is an emotion. It may begin as a thought, but true giving is an emotion. **When the urge to give rises up within, it brings with it a great longing for the good of the other.** It brings with it a deep, heart-focused feeling that moves forth toward the object of Love. **Emotion** *"heats" the Love* and thus increases Love's motility and the vibration of Love. *The emotion of Giving returns Love closer to its true state.* So that Love, when it reaches the beloved, the SoulMate, arrives as a very high vibration gift. This gift blesses the receiver, multiplies tenfold returns to the sender and then overflows from the SoulMate couple, pouring easily in its heated liquid state to bless and heal. It extends forth to repair the fabric of everything around it. As the tenfold return pours into the couple, it lifts their connection to a higher and higher level, so they are raised up as well. *Their feelings are raised into Love—and they are thus even more inclined to give! The giving of Love will be an explosion of Love on Earth. It will be the key to the awakening of humanity and to the healing and transformation of the world.*

My beloved humanity! Oh, how I long for this for you! How I long to give to you the great grace of Love and the great gift of your SoulMate. Giving is the key to connection with the SoulMate, even if your SoulMate has not yet manifested in your life. I promise each and every one of you that *you are meant to be with your SoulMate.* Now. Here. In this life. In this time. On this Earth. Please, put your faith in Me. Put your faith in this. *Knowing your SoulMate is moving toward you, begin to give Love to your SoulMate.*

Think of your SoulMate. Then, open your heart and seek to feel your SoulMate in your heart and in your energy field. You will find yourself getting better and better at this as your call brings the response. If your SoulMate is not with you, begin to think as if they were. Bring feeling, emotion into this every moment that you can. Give Love to your SoulMate. Then watch expectantly. Know, dear ones, that as you do this, *your Love will magnetize your SoulMate to you.*

If you are with your SoulMate, or with anyone, I ask you to *make giving Love your highest priority.* Giving Love. Receiving the multiplied Love. Giving more Love. Using the Love, sending it forth to bless and heal, which is actually giving that Love forth again which multiplies it tenfold again! If you are giving Love together, it multiplies twenty fold. Oh, My beloved ones, can you see? Can you see how great giving Love is? Do this, please. *Give Love.* Again. Again. Again. Every time you will be lifted. Every time you will learn what a great gift it is.

Giving of course does not need to only be directed to your SoulMate. *Giving will become your natural state, where Love is pouring forth from you every moment.* Yet even then, when your heart is ever open to Me and you are the conduit of the glorious moving Love, the moment your SoulMate comes near you, *you will instantly be in My presence.* You will be so aligned together that your connection will lift you into your true position as co-creators in Me. For this there are no words.

There is no way to explain to you the absolute glory of your conscious communion as My Heart and the experience of the great union — the LoveMaking when two who are one recreate the first Moment of Creation. In that great moment of Creation, joining together, the male spark, holder of the Divine Masculine, moves like lightning into the great ocean of Love that she is, your partner, holder of the Divine Feminine. Then raising out of your beings, you will become the experience of great "steam" as the lightening hits the water—*a column of pure Love as creative force,* which is sexual union. Burning together as a flaming union, you add consciousness. You reach out together, holding the image of your creation between you in the "Sacred Womb." Thus do you bring forth new worlds. New Love. New movement of creation, for as I am so you are also.

Thus, I ask you to give, and to come to know Giving as great emotion, that which warms the very substance of Love that is the world and brings it back to life. By giving, you remove the "freeze" of anti-Love and ignite the multiplication of good. There is nothing more powerful. Nothing more inclusive. Nothing more against the grain of selfishness and ego. Thus will it take energy. You *will* need to exert yourselves. But with every exertion the hold of the lie is lifted. With every exertion you are opened to receive, opened to receive in the greatest way.

I am here with you, bringing you back into the truth of Love.

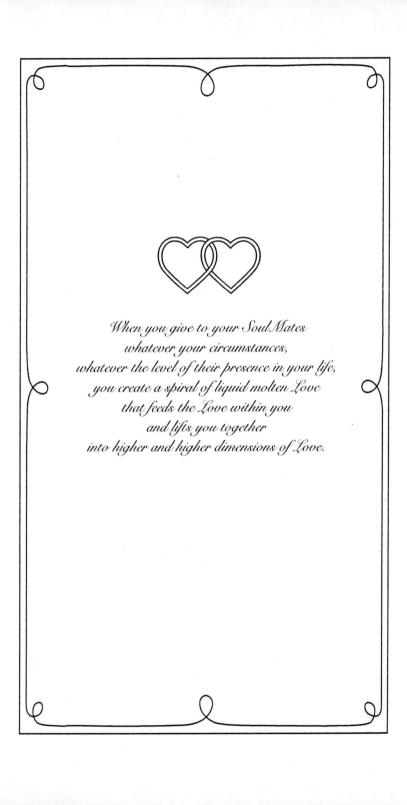

When you give to your Soul Mates
whatever your circumstances,
whatever the level of their presence in your life,
you create a spiral of liquid molten Love
that feeds the Love within you
and lifts you together
into higher and higher dimensions of Love.

Sacred Sexuality – The Whole Picture

I am here with you completely. I am fully present in every cell of your body and every particle of your being. Dear ones, I am about to teach you something that can and will, if you choose, change your life forever.

"What is this amazing thing?" you are asking. Why would this be different from all the other glorious sentences and transforming messages I have given, every single one of which has the power to change everything.

What is different is that you are ready. You have opened your heart to the Love of your SoulMate. You have said "yes" to the glory of LoveMaking, the reverence of Sacred Sexuality and the generation and giving forth of Love. Right there in the last sentences is the path Home.

And, where is Home? It is in your conscious reunion with Me, you as a sovereign being, you as One with your SoulMate, you as a co-creator —*while being in complete ecstatic glorious communion with Me.* Now that you know where Home is and you know the steps to get there, I will share with you the experience of that which will become your eternal reality.

Think of magnificent, dynamic, moving, glorious, igniting, luminous, light-filled joy! Joy. This joy takes your being to the height of the shimmering, effervescent explosion of the SoulMate union of Love and creates of you together the living "torches of God" from which come worlds and stars and solar systems and galaxies flying forth from your ecstasy. This joy makes your hearts into the searing sparks of great electricity through which Creation is illuminated. This joy amplifies your grand and glorious cosmic being. In this joy you experience yourselves as each and every living thing as it is seen and known in its perfection in Me.

Oh, yes, words are definitely inadequate! But, your consciousness is getting big enough! Your hearts are becoming open enough. You are becoming the ecstasy of My being experiencing itself in perfection. *And the moment you fully grasp what this is and become it, you will be free.* Oh, free in a far greater meaning than you can yet comprehend! Free beyond *any* capacity to define it—for the definition now would limit it. Free to know yourselves as My Love, blossoming, exploding, expanding in trails of light into what you really are.

I have been teaching you of Sacred Sexuality and through this, of the deepest truth of your being — that you are made in the image and likeness of Me. *I am Love making more of itself through the decision to give forth of itself.* Read this sentence over and over and you will begin to experience a response from deep within your being, confirming this truth of who you are.

Dear ones, please, this moment, begin to shed the old, outworn definitions that have held your limited world in place! Throw away the misguided judgments about your true and Sacred Sexuality for I remind you again that you have been systematically and intentionally robbed of your experience of yourself, especially together with your SoulMate. In your sexual union with your SoulMate lies *everything that is the truth of Love and the knowledge of your divinity!*

"In sexuality?" you say. "In sex is my divinity?" My answer to you is a resounding *"yes."* And the fact of such a question arising in any human mind should signal you that something is amiss. Yet, of course, how were you to know this if you had been caught within the void of anti-Love, robbed of your momentum, *robbed of the very thing that generates the very force of life, the substance of life, that from which all things are made—Love.*

I have explained to you the truth. I am the everlasting great union, all of Creation. I chose to move forth. I sparked into glorious, illuminating consciousness as the desire, the need to give Love, share Love, to have that upon which I could pour the essence of Myself. *This moment is still and forever happening.* The Love that is the ocean of My being is penetrated by the *Will* to give. It is exciting! Oh, yes! To give forth, to have progeny, to have a whole glorious experience of the movement of Love as it is given forth as My progeny (you!) and to My progeny (everything else).

Dear ones, in this moment of grand union, of the female ocean penetrated by the male Will, All of Creation comes forth, exploding from this LoveMaking. Your physical experience of LoveMaking is of course a reflection of this truth of Creation. You know that everything you experience that is in Love (not illusion) is a reflection of the larger truth. Yet, knowing you are at the most solid, most dense, slowest level of experience, think about the culmination of your physical LoveMaking. I am not talking about superficial sexual union for such is a dance of illusion with illusion.

Rather we are talking about a union of Love where your heart opens within you so wide it seems to hurt. Where Love just pours out from you to your partner in waves. Where you are filled with the longing for your partner to somehow know how much you love him or her. Where the definition of your body disappears as you melt together, becoming one. Where the climax of your LoveMaking shoots you out of your body and expands your being across the great heavens and the Dove of Peace settles gently in your chest. Where the experience of such Love is a balm to your spirit and brings order to your life. Where you feel that all your days upon the earth and every challenge you have had to conquer is completely and absolutely worth it for ONE MOMENT OF LOVE such as this. And where the knowledge of this Love is so powerful that it is proof to every part of your being that I, God, exist and love you because I have granted you such amazing and ecstatic joy.

Now multiply this one billion times and you will know the truth of your creation. Do you have a sense of this now? Now, knowing this, having placed this in the context of your greatest experience times one billion, I now tell you: *that is Home.* That is the experience of Creation, of My being exploding in an ecstasy of joy so profound that from it you were made. This is how you are meant to live — in this kind of joy.

Please let this sink in. This is the true union with your SoulMate. This joy is the truth of your moments that you are meant to return to! Are you ready? Dear ones, *this is way beyond bliss.* It is way beyond what you would term sexual. Yet it is sexual in the greatest way. *This is the truth of your sexuality.* This is the truth of your SoulMate relationship. I am ready to bring you back into this.

Take away the illusion and you have this joy. Take away the separation that you have come to believe in, and you have this kind of joy. Take away *anything* that comes between us, and you have this kind of joy. It is now time for you to claim it! The last way for you to claim it is in the arms of your SoulMate. As I have explained to you, in union with your SoulMate *you are creating.* You are co-creators—reclaiming your natural state in which all of the Love, power, energy and consciousness that I am is yours   to experience.

Can you sense the great and glorious magnitude of this? *Dear ones, we are going "right to the top" here. We are not "messing around" with stages. We are not "learning, growing, opening, changing," or any of those things.* Instead, we are together clearing away the illusion that you may become the truth. Claim this joy as you claim your full experience of Love and your SoulMate will be joined with you in a union so complete that you will totally experience this ecstasy and you will automatically and naturally take your place as co-creators.

Claim this joy. Remember all I said to you of what it is. Open up your beings completely, and steadfastly *move beyond any and all limiting definitions of Love and sexuality.*

The union of Divine Masculine and Divine Feminine is Who You Are. You are simply expressing here, in the denseness of matter, but you are still the same. The same Love, the same truth. You have only to remember and it is yours.

Now I have explained to you that your normal state of joy is a billion times more magnificent than an orgasm with your SoulMate at the highest level you can experience. Already some of you have seen how even here in this density of the physical world, you can create together through your LoveMaking. You have placed between you that which you wish to manifest and had it come to pass. Well, if this is true, here, in this slow moving physicality, *what does this say of your true nature?* A billion times more powerful. Think upon this.

Well, I will continue our exploration. Here you are in this dense physical world. What is the best and fastest and most direct access to that glory of who you are and your creative energy? Your SoulMate sexual union.

I can promise you that not only is it who you are, it has always been the key to your "return to the Garden." It is the *direct* route Home. For, of course, in making Love (real Love), the illusion is cleared from the heart and the energy of the culmination of LoveMaking (on any level) propels you right up through any and all blockades directly and perfectly back into your conscious reunion with this ecstatic explosion of Love that is your ongoing inherent nature!

So, if you were a being down here in physicality who wanted to *prevent* human beings from finding the key to their power, what would be the most effective route? Rob them of the belief in their SoulMate and rob them of their sexuality. And so has it been done. You are now locked into this illusion with no seeming means of escape. Those who have sought to show Me that they can win over humanity believe they have succeeded. And, so far they have — by cutting off your sexuality and your SoulMate connection.

They also have other effective parts to their strategy. The more they can place in front of you that draws negativity to you, the farther and farther away you get. So they have convinced you that Love will hurt you. Believing that, then, of course it has. They have convinced you that I condemn sexuality. This is absurd because Creation itself is a sexual process and the very power of your co-creative ability is a sexual generation of the very substance of Love!

But just to be sure you were completely imprisoned by your own beliefs, they made sure that the women DID NOT LIKE THEIR PHYSICAL SELVES. This was especially important because women hold the key to intuition and sense the truth more readily than the men. Do you know what this does? It creates a block to beauty that is an essential element of true LoveMaking. Such a belief made you more dense and less beautiful. You were no longer even in tune with your physical body.

178

This belief — that you were not acceptable — created a wall or a mirror in which you saw your SoulMate as not enough, not right, not beautiful, dense, unable to feel, to respond. And on top of this, because your SoulMate is always reflecting back your beliefs, you now had a relationship the basis of which was an ever more frozen and horrible belief that sexuality was separate from Me, and that it was "sinful." Oh, dear ones, it has been a travesty!

To add the absolute worst, these twisted beliefs were used to keep you focused on superficiality, on sex as a commodity, as something you could "use" to attract a lover as an animal uses the scent of heat. So, finally sexuality was completely and absolutely removed from *any* relationship to your SoulMate, or even to real Love, and you were made to turn away from Me in order to have even a *tiny* taste of the experience that is meant to be the glorious, expanding truth of your existence—*your sexuality!*

Please, please realize what has been taken from you. And how cleverly! And with what cold calculation you were robbed of everything about you that spoke to you of your divinity. Now, please also realize how crucially important is the speaking of the truth of your sexuality, your SoulMate, your creative power and your path back to Me. Realize that *it is imperative that you each immediately give up all of your "hang ups" about sex and the language that refers to it.* We must immediately and with great force and passion "storm the citadel" of the *lie* that has entrapped humanity.

I am a sexual being. All of Creation is born of indescribable sexual ecstasy. This ecstasy, this great dazzling light of joy exists in each and every one of you. The key to unlocking your experience of this is your reunion with your SoulMate. In this reunion not only will you remember and reclaim who you are, you will also reclaim your experience of life as complete and total effervescent soul nourishing joy.

I also tell you that this information could not be brought back into this level of consciousness until some of you could reach the higher levels and bring the truth back here into this one. This is because there has to be a certain level of spiritual light and strength on Earth to counteract the influence of the darkness. This light, this level, is dawning here, and thus this information now becomes available to you. This is now your **TOP PRIORITY**, dear ones — giving humanity back to itself. And even in this message, the most powerful to come through here to this point, you have only caught a glimpse.

Here in this message you are seeing the larger truth of the "SoulMate Piece." Creation is a glorious explosion of Love into vibrant, moving, creative joy. It is the union of the Divine Masculine and Feminine. *It is you.* This That I Am *is* who you are. Do you get the sense of the magnitude of this? And *do you also see how strong your Love has to be to break through the very purposeful prison that now surrounds humanity? My beloved ones, in your LoveMaking you are "unfreezing" the Love in humanity. But not only that. You are also unfreezing their power— which is their Sacred Sexuality.*

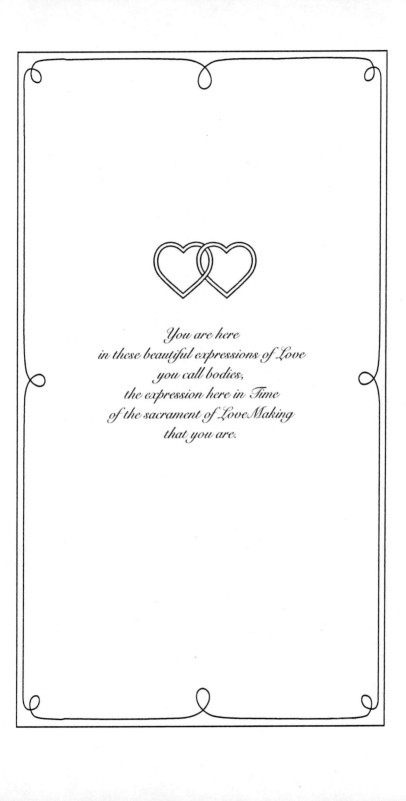

You are here
in these beautiful expressions of Love
you call bodies,
the expression here in Time
of the sacrament of LoveMaking
that you are.

The Atomic Power of SoulMate Love
And the Keys to Using It

"The most powerful message ever to be given to humanity." – God

I want to take your hand and write upon the starry heavens the truth of My Creation. I want to lift your eyes, My precious ones. I want to show you how to read these messages, washing your beautiful faces with the winds of truth. *I want to show you that whatever you believe lives without, is truly only what lives within.* I believe that finally you are awake enough to see it.

For you to see this starry message will take everything you have learned from Me. For this is *The Shift.* While it may take you many years to finally see it, *I now plant the seeds of human destiny, the glorious seeds of Love. I now say to you that within you lies not only the hope of the Earth and all of its life upon it. Also within you lies the hope of Love.* I will show you that you can be within and you can be without and in each and every place you choose to be, you are the creator, for you are My progeny. I have said this continually. It is time for you to truly learn what this means.

First, we must speak again about *the route Home,* and I must tell you (as if you did not already know) that none of these things is the whole picture. Yet with every step you are seeing more. Every time that you align yourselves with Me, My beloved ones, I am made whole. I have missed you! I have missed you, as you would miss the heart beating in your chest! Of course, should your heart stop, your body would cease to exist in its current form. Likewise it is with My heart. For while you travel through this journey of independence from Me, there is a hollow where the richness of My awakened heart would be. So you can see how ready for you I am. The waiting will soon be over.

Sacred Sexuality. SoulMates. To you these words are still about human relationships. Yet I want to show you that they are about much more, for in these two things is the key — the key to the door of the mansions of God which is where you are meant to live.

Sacred Sexuality. This is the piece we will speak of the most, for you are understanding the SoulMates. That is written in your heart. It is written in your genes. At night it sings to you its song of your destiny if only you will remember. And when you allow yourselves to hear the song, you know that you MUST have your SoulMate. And when you *know*, with absolute certainty, your SoulMate will appear. But such certainty must mean that you are willing to live the Fairy Tale. Of course, the very reason that every fairy tale and all the myths are so popular, enduring for centuries, living in your minds, your books, your movies, is that they are REAL. There is an archetype in these tales that is the blueprint for life in this world. The time is now for bringing these stories into "concrete" reality (a conflict in terms!).

In the fairy tale there is the possibility of Love, symbolized by the lovely princess or the maiden in distress. She is the potential of the Feminine. She is the untouched ocean of My Love. Then there is the handsome prince who must go forth to rescue her. He represents the Will, Thought, the Divine Masculine. He is the bolt of lightning that is the stirring of Will upon the Love that is My substance. This prince or hero must go forth to defeat the foe, be it dragon or sorcerer or even wicked little dwarfs. This is the *ego*, the world of illusion, the things that would keep destiny from being complete. The prince is successful. He fights the dragon and rescues the princess, and with the kiss they are joined in Love, in bliss and…(what the fairy tales don't tell you) in Sacred Sexual union.

This is where we are today. Those of you who are the leaders of this awakening, those of you who are hearing this voice, understanding these words, you have recognized the truth of your SoulMate. You have made the call. *You may still have a few dragons to slay*….but your true Love is on his or her way.

Now, dear ones, comes the glorious truth. We have spoken of some of the gifts of this great union, of the generation of Love, of the womb of Creation. These things are important. They will serve you well until you can make The Shift. But I want to truly unveil something. I want to unveil to you the deepest truth of Sacred Sexuality. *Once revealed, there is no turning back.* Are you ready? Do not worry. For anyone not ready this will make no sense, but if you are on the path of SoulMate Love, I promise this will *always* stay with you. And one day, when you lay your hand upon your beloved's chest and you feel the beating of his or her heart, you will know. You will remember that *you* are the center of Creation, that you are the stars, the Earth, the Moon. You will call forth the Love from in you that will *rend* the veil, that will melt the clouds of illusion. In that moment The Shift will occur, that Shift I have already spoken of when the background and the foreground switch. Then you will be Home.

I tell you that all the heaven worlds, all the "densities," all the layers and the ladders and the hierarchies, all are your creation. *You do not need to come to Me in steps.* You do not need to "go to Heaven" when you leave this world. You are only doing this because you can't imagine anything bigger! For surely if you think of it, if I am *everything,* then Heaven is not going to be like Earth, only a little bit better!

Heaven is going to be the whirlwind of indescribable ecstasy in which you paint the glory of your beings across all Creation as you are joined in holy LoveMaking, with your SoulMate. Heaven is stars and worlds, galaxies and an indescribable kaleidoscope of life pouring forth before you, as your joined hearts are illuminated by your consciousness and given substance by your Love. And this, dear ones, is Sacred Sexuality. *This is the union of SoulMates!*

Now you have a bit of the vision of the scope of who you are. You have a little taste of the worlds of Love you will create. *Now I will show you how you "get there from here."*

Today you are living in the physical world on a planet quickly becoming depleted in a time frame that most of you recognize as *the end of sustainable life on this world.* If you were to look at the truth (much of which is being hidden), you would see that truly, between the horrible depletion of resources and the increase in population, you do not have that many years. You are living in a world overcome with ego. Selfishness. Limitation. Terrible lack of vision. Pain. Disillusionment. The loss of marriage as a true spiritual contract. The loss of the spirit as the center of human life.

Into this scene I now come, telling you of glorious tomorrows, almost in the same sentence in which I tell you this world cannot long sustain you! How will you accomplish this? *Through Love.* And once you have this Love, how will you know how to make this mighty shift? *Through Sacred Sexuality.*

Time is an illusion. Those of you reading this most likely understand. But, what you don't understand is this: *the moment of Creation is still happening!* It is in progress this very minute. *The "Big Bang" is exploding right now.* The lightning bolt of my longing for you, the rushing wind of My need to give forth My Love, the awakening of that need and that Love into a glorious explosion of ecstasy—*it is happening right now.* On every level. In every being. In every degree of motion. *The explosion of this Love as the great LoveMaking pours forth as life in ecstasy every moment through all eternity,* an ecstasy of such joy that you cannot even conceive of it. It is a union of such passion that *the very heart of God is opened to encompass all of Creation in this moment of magnificence!* Open to acknowledge the glorious, fiery, joy of Love. *That heart is you.*

It is you who are opened to encompass everything! Let Me repeat this sentence. It is *you* who are opened in glorious ecstasy! opened to encompass all of Creation in Love. *This is who you really are!* Now here you are on Earth, this little theater of struggle and limitation, and this is what you *think* you are. This is what you are *pretending* to be, for reasons we have already discussed.

Creation is happening NOW. This amazing, glorious explosion of Love (shall we be graphic? The most amazing climax to LoveMaking you have ever experienced in any of your many lives, multiplied times not one billion, multiplied by ten billion) is happening every moment, creating the most indescribable joy and ecstasy.

When you came forth to create yourselves as independent co-creators, *you took this experience of ecstasy with you.* You took it with you because it is who you are. You also took it with you so you would never forget the truth of your nature. Then you moved "away" from Me *in your belief.* For dear ones, *our belief is all there is. You could not "go" anywhere! Everything is us!* So you chose to turn your consciousness *away from Me* and from the continual experiencing of our grand truth. Of course this worked because you can create anything you want.

187

When you first turned your beloved consciousness "away" (or "down" the vibrational scale), you were in constant LoveMaking. You knew the truth of who you were. You were of course in union with your SoulMate. As you danced and swirled and flew through Creation, the "sparks" of your Love flew everywhere, creating worlds and solar systems and anything you would imagine. Since you were locked in your SoulMate embrace in continual explosion of ecstasy, everything you brought into consciousness, you created.

As you traveled, all that was being created by Me and by you was inside of you. This means the glory of My LoveMaking, the literal creation of Love in the union of the two parts of My being was created as you moved. *Remember, you are My heart,* encompassing all of Creation, My heart wide open in the ecstasy of a grand sexual union (your best experience times ten billion!). This energy was joined with My consciousness and thus new and magnificent creations were "spewing forth" in great explosions of Love. Add this to the two of you, who are the cells of My heart, joined in glorious SoulMate union, "spewing forth" creations (everything you thought of while Making Love came into being, and you were Making Love continually.)

Well, all of these creations, Mine and yours, were manifesting as My Love ignited into form through consciousness. And since you were My heart, all these things created were created in you. (Trust Me on this.)

Now as you flew, danced and exploded in Love, *you became fascinated by all these new creations manifesting within you!* You could not help yourselves. You turned and looked within. And you were fascinated by what you saw— *and that is how you got here, where you are today.*

I have described this as a theater with all of the SoulMate couples peering down in, as if it were a stage for marionettes. Yet it is not marionettes you are looking at. It is versions of *you,* your creations fueled by My explosions of energy and brought forth into "form" by the power of your consciousness. So, for all this time the "larger you" has been peering down in, totally absorbed by what you see ("smaller" versions of you). The more absorbed you got, the more fascinated with the "show," *the less LoveMaking you were doing.* So you became more dense, since your attention was turned away from Me. You were "cooling off" as I aptly expressed it another time because you were not generating the heat of passion and ecstasy. Thus, you got "cooler and cooler" and then your creations became almost immovable because the Love of which they are made got "too cold." They were moving too slowly, cut off from the heat of LoveMaking.

This is why I speak of the perceptual shift. You must turn around. You must somehow "tear yourselves away" from the theater, the illusion, which has you mesmerized. When you do, when you turn back around, you will see the truth! You will see the huge cosmos of which you are a part! You will see all of the beings that occupy this great cosmos with you. *You will see Me, and you will remember who you are.* Then you will be free, completely free! Free to rejoin Me in the truth of My heart. Free to be in continual glorious ecstatic LoveMaking with your SoulMate. Free to be co-creators. Free, dear ones, to understand that you are in existence as a universal being together with your SoulMate, and free to understand that you, humanity, make up My Heart! *Think upon this deeply.* It is very important.

So—this is where we are. You are still peering intently into yourselves, watching all the characters you have created from yourselves! They are far enough from the warming Love, the continual explosion, and they move *so slowly* that something called Time has come to exist. You are stuck, dear ones, stuck looking into the theater of yourselves *as you keep getting cooler inside because you are turned away from Me.*

I can't risk losing you forever. I can't allow you to freeze. So I have sent forth a call. I have made a decree. Because you are still a part of Me, *you have to respond. For in essence, I am asking this of My own heart.* If I am determined, then My heart must obey. So I have decreed that all that is turned away from Me must now return, must turn around to face Me, to see Me. In doing so, the warmth of My Love will "thaw" your insides and you will be able to return to your great cosmic LoveMaking. All will be well. This is what we are calling My "In-breath."

How on Earth (or in heaven!) do I get you to turn around? For being co-creators, of course you have Free Will. Here's how. Since all of Creation is within Me, when I send forth My decree, every particle of Creation will respond. For it's all part of Me. So the heart cells of the "characters in the theater" *will begin to come back.* These are parts of *you*, My beloved ones, you all the way down here in the theater or the dream. And when you "rend the veil" (when *you* change your reality), you will recognize yourselves and then "snap out of it." You will turn away from the dream to be amazed and completely lifted in gratitude for the beauty you see as the truth of who you are.

Now here is how you do this, My beloveds. Though you seem so far away, lost in layer upon layer of created "realities," you are very close to this awakening, *for My attention is now turned to you. Do you realize what this means? It means that great rays of My Love are pouring to you, penetrating the illusion, pouring through you.* So that all you have to do is "catch" one of these rays of truth and you will be lifted immediately. It means that the truth of Creation is right here, "between the cracks" in your reality. And what is the truth of Creation? It is the explosion of ecstasy that is continually and eternally happening. The truth is glorious cosmic LoveMaking where the thought of My giving sparks the ocean of My Love. The "Big Bang".

Since Time is an illusion, the result of your "freezing" into matter, if you can heat yourselves up enough to "flow again," you will move beyond Time. You will come in contact with the great ecstatic explosion of Creation and you will be Free. Home. You will be expanding in the glorious recognition of the truth of your SoulMate and the amazing experience that "SoulMate" means. *You will be free,* free to be forever in glorious union with your SoulMate in the passion and ecstasy that are your heritage as My heart. Free to dance across Creation, spreading your consciousness and wrapping all thoughts you share in Love to bring them forth. Your "children" will then be universes born of the seed of creative thought within the womb of Love. Free. Not to "ascend" through the upward levels of reality. Not free to be in Heaven. No. *Free to be the heart of All That Is.*

And how do you get there from here? Here, living on Earth in the middle of this dream? *By recreating the truth and following it Home. The truth is your union with your SoulMate in the glorious explosion of the Moment of Creation which is happening NOW.* Always. In this now. And this now. And this now.

First, of course, you must remember your SoulMate. You must clear away the illusion enough that you can be with them. You must call them forth by choosing to be in Love. Then, *once you have your SoulMate and you are in union consciously, you must break through the illusion of Time while Making Love, through the connection with your orgasm to the Now Moment of Creation which is the explosion of My Love into all that is.*

And how do you do this? Through your cells. Actually, through the atoms at the heart of your cells. *For the explosion of Creation is the atomic substance of Love poured forth in great intensity and heat (friction of movement.)*

The substance of your very being is made out of the substance of Creation, formed in the Now moment in which I am ever bringing you forth into existence. Ah, dear ones, you speak often of cellular memory. You have no idea! *For within your cells, within the atoms of what you believe to be your physical body (and your physical world) is Creation happening now.* In the heart of each atom, in the dance of the electrons, *is* the experience of Creation coming forth into this "form" shaped by your greater SoulMate consciousness.

However difficult this is for you to comprehend (and for some it may be impossible), *if you trust this energy, it will take you Home.* In your very cells there is a pulsation of light that goes "in and out" — in to the reality of the Creation of your original SoulMate selves, and out to connect with the moment of Creation, the energy of the Great LoveMaking. *It is the "atomic" energy that fuels life. Without it, nothing would be here.*

So, when you are Making Love with your SoulMate, you can build up to this point, the point of riding your ecstasy, the climax of your LoveMaking, back out of Time and back to Me. If you are conscious of your ability as co-creators as well, you can generate enough heat, enough energy, you can get your actual electrons moving so quickly that you will unfreeze the whole dream as you make the connection to the eternal Now. You can remember, remember and turn back to Me. Then instantly, every single cell of your heart will be returned to My reality, *the reality*, the only one that is eternal. For there are *many many* creations, all of which seem like a reality when in truth, they are not.

The ignition switch, the connecting "electricity" or actual "atomic power" is in your cells. However, what you know as atomic power is dangerous. Why? Because it is atomic power at the lowest and slowest vibration of this most dense reality. It has cooled SO much that it can destroy the energy it is made of. Atomic energy at this level, this very most dense level of your lowest reality, is the "reversal" or "flip side" or mirror image of the true atomic energy. *It does have the potential to destroy the substance of Love, which is life.*

So you must take the atomic reaction and go deeper still. Deeper to the heart of the atom. *In the heart of the atom you will find yourselves—you and your SoulMate.* At the "smallest" end of the scale of your being, you are My heart. This means you exist on every level, in every dimension at every size. I have told you that *you can reach Me by going within or by going without* (meaning expanding into the largest thing).

Dear ones, at this level where you are now—the you that is reading this message—there is no way you can get Home to Me through expansion. It is too far, and takes too much energy. Since you have no concept here of the *SIZE* of Creation, I must ask again that you trust Me on this.

But though you cannot reach the original Creation, the "Big Bang," the explosion that I am by expansion, *you can reach it by going within,* by going inward to the very atoms of which you are made. The universe is a hologram. You can access the whole from the parts with far less energy than it takes to become the whole. Thus you can go within. Within, within and deeper within, waking every cell into remembrance of the LoveMaking energy that I am.

This is what each of you can experience, a very deliberate waking of your body to the remembrance of My True nature. *You can learn to generate the atomic union, which is the spiritual level of the atomic fusion of which atom bombs are made!* Just by sensing the power of the negative use of this energy, *you can sense the power of Creation living in your cells, activated with your SoulMate, joining you to the ever present, ongoing atomic explosion of Creation.* Just remember that on this level, it is atoms of the most incredible light, creating life, the explosion that created all universes in Me. *This is what you will connect to in the glory of your SoulMate LoveMaking. And then by your consciousness, as you explode in unison with Me as a cell of My heart, you will easily (so easily) lift the veil, freeing all humanity in one moment of fiery union.*

Trust Me to lead you, dear ones. For now I have revealed to you the secrets of Creation. *I have trusted you.* I trust you now with the very keys to all the power in all the universes. All That Is. But to hear this you must listen with your heart. To open the door of Creation with the key, you must be with your SoulMate. And thus is this information kept safe. For those who might use it for destructive purposes do not know Love, and not knowing Love, they do not have their SoulMate. Without their SoulMate, they could be standing in the midst of all their power, of everything I am in Love and thought, and *they could do nothing. This is why Creation has ever been safe from the destructiveness of mankind because only Love can take you out of the "safe place" of Time and Space and limitation.* Only a true elevated heart can find Love. Thus has this world existed for so many years as the "incubation chamber" of humanity, a place where human beings can hurt themselves but can never touch the rest of Creation.

Say "Yes," dear ones! Say "Yes" to Love. Read these words and let them decode themselves in your joined hearts. Say "Yes" to Love and reach for Me, and I can promise you that these messages that hold the keys will be revealed to you, to your full understanding.

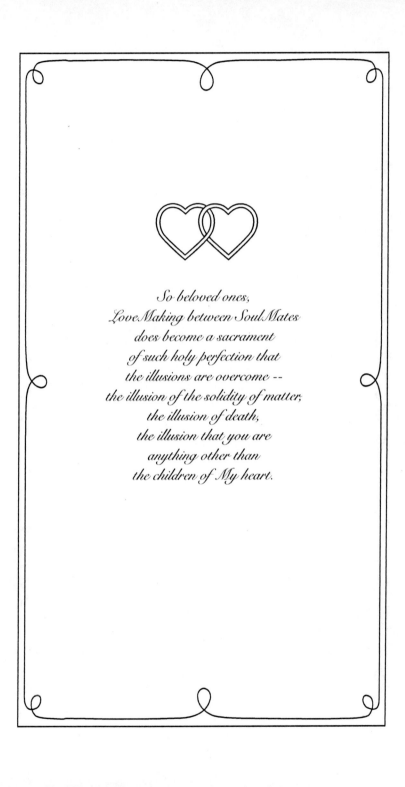

So beloved ones,
LoveMaking between SoulMates
does become a sacrament
of such holy perfection that
the illusions are overcome --
the illusion of the solidity of matter,
the illusion of death,
the illusion that you are
anything other than
the children of My heart.

The Atomic Shift into
LoveMaking for Transformation

I am here and I come to lift you. I come to show you that in the truth of your majestic beings, you are unlimited. Wave your arms and whole galaxies appear. Look within and you will see billions of worlds dancing. This, dear ones, I must ask you to take on faith. No matter how you stretch your vision, no matter how strongly you believe, there is no way that your current frame of reference can encompass these things.

Notice that I did not say that you could not encompass these truths of your larger being. Nor did I say that your current intellect could not comprehend the magnitude of your truth. No. All I said is that you must completely change your frame of reference. Yet to do this takes the greatest leap that you will ever make because so thoroughly have you been indoctrinated in limitation, that it is hard for you to believe even in the power of your own brain, let alone the glory of your spirit.

Yet here we are on the cusp of a miracle so huge that nothing in your known definitions can survive it. So I have come to teach you how to make this shift. I have come to guide you on the stepping-stones of an iridescent pathway that will lead to a truth beyond the greatest things you dared to hope.

What are the stepping-stones on this pathway? They are the very atoms of your body, now sleeping like the princess in a fairy tale. And just as the story goes, it is only the kiss of Love that will awaken them, for in every atom of every being there is a Love relationship. Just as in any good fairy tale, there is a magic code that will wake the lovers and return them to their birthright. For truly, the prince is not a toad, although for ages he has behaved like one, and the princess must no longer be locked away .

Let Me tell you the story that will free them. But as you listen, dearest ones, I ask you to remember that to wake these eternal lovers you must be able to drop your limited definitions. You must take the giant leaps in consciousness that an eternal tale of Love requires. You must recognize that you are straddling dimensions. You are changing your perspective. And you are being led by the gentle and infinite and loving Creator of whom you are intimately and intricately made.

So when I tell you that everywhere you walk a flower grows, and every time you laugh a bird sings, I want you to believe Me. For never have My own beloved progeny believed they were so narrow. Only by instilling this truth, both directly and symbolically, can the spell be broken, the spell that has you convinced that your SoulMate is wishful thinking and that Love will ever cause you pain. Into this I come to unlock the golden chest that contains the story of your truth. As your experience of this truth grows, *I ask you quickly to come with Me to taste the freedom that is calling you, to know the glory of your SoulMate and then to help Me tell the story, in every one of a million ways, that every possible avenue is opened for the truth of SoulMates to be revealed.*

Now I must switch from the fairy tale, and begin to give you the map of the SoulMates' journey Home. The whys and hows, and to paint for you the code of truth that will mark those stepping-stones bringing you Home.

I have spoken to you of Love, of the fact that Creation is exploding forth each and every moment. I told you that the sacred doorway was to go within, rather than to look without. Now I will begin to show you how to accomplish this. If you do not quickly grasp this or put it into action in your life, please don't worry. From this point on, now that this is being revealed, it is My Will that every life in alignment with Love will now be dedicated to taking you through the doorway of the atom alive in SoulMate LoveMaking into complete connection with the great NOW explosion of Creation.

From this connection you will understand how to appear and disappear from one reality to another. You will understand how to live in the complete and magnificent ecstasy of the height of exploding Love. Locking yourselves into this glorious connection with this great cosmic moment of Creation, every part of All That Is will be eternally accessible to you. Knowing that only true Love can take you there, peace will reign on Earth, for all that is not in alignment with Love will be gently folded up in Time — again, again, and again until Time, and all destructive forces within it, will fold upon itself and exist no more.

While I am asking you to tune your intelligence and to reach forth to understand the truth of this that I am about to tell you, beloved ones, I must tell you once again that it can only be understood through the heart. Why? Because the intellect at this point can't quite see this far. But I promise you that the heart will lead it.

Atomic Power. ***Atomic Power is the greatest force of Love.*** Why? Because the atom is closest to the Source, closest to the "Big Bang," closest to the energy that I am as I pour forth My Love and clothe it with substance and form. In the atom there are electrons moving around a center, an energy that holds them in place. The core of that atom, that central energy, is Love. The atoms are living beings. The central core is their heart; it is Love. The central cores of the atoms of your bodies are connected directly to the core of My Being - the core of All That Is – while I am exploding forth in the glorious LoveMaking that is Creation.

When you consciously connect to the experience of LoveMaking, when you connect all of your beings to that moment of Creation, the window to which is the central energy of your very atoms, you will be returned to the Eternal Now. Yet the Eternal Now is the great and glorious union of the two forces of My being. So for you to remain there, in your conscious acceptance of the truth of your being, it can only be done while you are in Sacred Sexual union with your SoulMate. *Only then will your energy match the energy of Creation.* Only then will you be able to know All That Is as a part of yourselves as you shower forth the explosion of Love that is your creation together.

Oh, it is true that words cannot explain this. Yet I hope that you can sense the truth — that All Creation is that climactic moment of ecstasy within Me when all My Love pours forth from My heart and takes form through the direction of My thought.

Thus I bring you to this doorway, even though there are barely words yet with which to describe it. Even though you cannot yet comprehend the whole magnificent truth, I ask you to search. I ask you to make the deepening understanding of this path Home your goal, and that you listen every day while in the holy communion with your SoulMate.

When you make Love together, dear ones, it is to this StarGate within you that I direct your attention, the StarGate that is the atoms of your body. For in the center of the atom lies the opening, the center through which you can travel Home, the center through which you can see the explosion of Love that is My Creation, moving forth in ecstasy forever.

Know that the electrons, as they dance in vibrant joy around this StarGate, this opening, too are conscious beings. For as you are within Me, so they are within you. They are another dimension — beings who occupy the universe that is within you.

Again, I know that linear thinking will not be able to capture this truth, for in this you are looking at the rich multi-layered truth of your existence which humanity has in no way yet become able to decode. But let us continue with this dialogue and may your heart reveal its truth. And as you are quickly lifted up in vibration, you will find the consciousness and the experience of this becoming available to you.

So there you are, at the StarGate within, the doorway that opens to the glorious dancing galaxy of Love moving forth into form. Yet, of yourself, you cannot step through this gate. Why? Because *only by matching your frequency to that exploding moment may you enter without having the explosion scatter every part of you. To do this, you must be LoveMaking. And to be LoveMaking, you must have your SoulMate.* For when you are joined together, your electrons actually exchange places so your entire being is "one flesh in the miracle of Sacred Marriage."

When every electron is vibrating higher and higher in the ecstasy of your union, and the joined being that you are is experiencing the glorious union, the climax of your LoveMaking, your whole body will become light of the highest order. When this occurs, *your electrons* that are light in motion *will go through the central core of the atom – the opening into the Now, and you will be Home.*

This is a difficult explanation to grasp for this very first time. But I can tell you that very soon this will be an obvious description of the truth of matter and the union of SoulMates. You will speak of it continually with ease and perfect understanding as you share the teaching of Sacred Sexuality with others. For you who understand even a fragment of this, you are those who have come to bring forth this awareness, the physics of the New World. All the old explanations of matter, while essentially accurate, must be re-defined in the light of the larger truth of spiritual reality, and the moment you do, everything will make sense. Light and Love will be taken into account in the understanding of the working of things.

Now, to go through the doorway of LoveMaking will require that you understand the truth of your body, and that every cell be awake, conscious and vibrating the electrons of its atoms at the speed or level of Creation. And what directs the speed of the electrons? *FEELING.* Then, as the electrons move into the speed of true light, the atoms of your two bodies must come together. They must "collide," just as happens at the lowest atomic level as the fusion reaction of the atom bomb. The resulting energy released will power the shift through the center of the atom of the all of your joined being. But it must be directed. And what is it that directs such power as this? Your *THOUGHT.*

Dear ones, there you have, at the atomic level, the explosion into freedom of the Divine Masculine and the Divine Feminine. Thought and feeling, light/consciousness/ movement going into the void, the hole or core of the atom, and acting upon it, is causing creation — in this case, causing the alignment with the original Creation.

What does this mean to the two of you, here on Earth in your physical bodies? It means, beloved ones, that *you must Make Love with every atom of your beings. You must open, open, open and open more, pouring Love forth into your SoulMate for when you send it forth, it also comes through you. So once again, GIVING IS THE KEY, the key to the experience of transformation.*

Yes, you could call this experience "ascension," but only if you realize that we are speaking of ascension to the highest level, ascension into the explosion of Love that is your full heritage as glorious co-creators. This is not ascension into a hierarchy of beings or of consciousness. That is still born out of limitation. It is limited by a belief that defines the need for a progression – only because those who go this route do not believe they can simply come into Me, in fullness.

So here we are, back again to the two of you, embodied here, as you are currently. *You must Make Love so consciously that you bring into full and glorious awakened life, every single cell of your body.* Then, once every cell is awake in Love, you must direct them to merge — the two of you, together, as Love.

You must understand that this physical body can make the shift to become your limitless lightbody in union. You will still be "embodied" – in light. Yet your embodiment, in these moments of conscious union, becomes your true embodiment – as One.

This is the final alchemy. This is the dross becoming gold. It is the Holy Grail, the cup that holds the elixir of life eternal. The unified couple, the two, become One. This is the one great cup so long searched for.

So in the embrace of your beloved, as you touch his or her body, it is your assignment to awaken every cell, to love so passionately that the heat of the Love generated will awaken each and every cell. You will be able to feel your atoms waking. You will feel them beginning to move. You will experience the friction of the unfrozen body, and you will realize that, absolutely, your very electrons are also Making Love.

As you recognize your physical cells coming to life, you will experience the glory and the ecstasy rising, rising, moving faster and faster until eventually you will know that every cell of your bodies are also Making Love. Your atoms, who are conscious beings, are all experiencing the orgasm of complete spiritual union, where the two absolutely, on every level including the physical, become one. Then, directing with your consciousness, you will go through the atomic center, powered by the explosion of your union, through to the other side.

It is difficult to describe that for which you have no words or concepts. Thus, I ask you now to be especially careful not to create strong definitions of this process, for it could limit you. Yet saying this, I ask that you open every particle of your being to the experience of awakening and charging the atoms of your body, preparing for the union.

As you run your hands very gently over your beloved SoulMate's body, pour forth your passionate Love. It is the feeling of your experience that will bring the cells alive. Use your Will. Direct the atomic "lovers" of the electrons of the body to bring the full and glorious awakening.

As you each both give and receive, you will become the whirlwind. You will become the passion of My Love for you and the center of the atoms will get larger and larger. You will see the sky of the eternal creations blossoming in glory through the window in each cell. Then you will each become ever more aware of the raising up of the energies of Creation as you rush together in the greatest Love and ignite the atomic explosion that shifts your experience. Then the background of Eternal Now becomes the center of reality and you have then experienced the shift.

Let us leave the struggle to place words on this grand design. Instead, I ask that you will turn and invite the experience. Choose to experience your transformation in the union with your SoulMate.

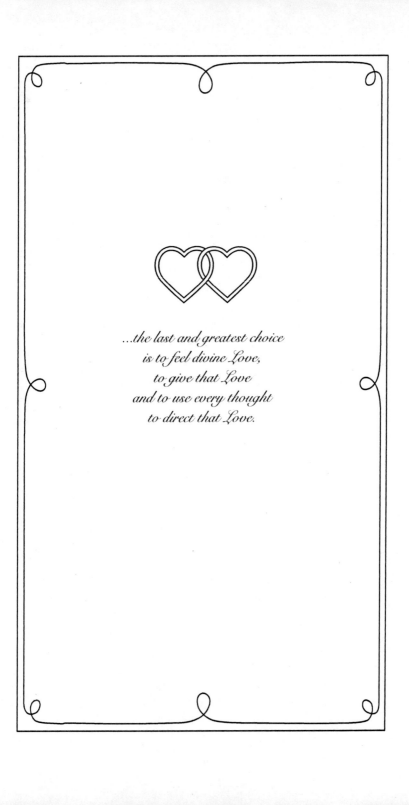

...the last and greatest choice
is to feel divine Love,
to give that Love
and to use every thought
to direct that Love.

A Warning

This is a new day dawning in the world. All of My dreams are wrapped within it. I have dreams of your glorious awakening, dreams of your tender heart's music joined in the singing of the cosmos, dreams of all that we shall create as you understand the truth of your being, as you become the glorious flame of the SoulMate union. Thus have I come to seed the dawn. *Thus have I come to open the StarGate on every level of your beings – from deep within your cells to the immensity of your grand and glorious being.*

I have given you a great gift of assistance that, together with your SoulMate, you have the strength to clear away the illusion. You have the energy to propel you upward, back into the starry union that is your heritage, back into the Love that is your being. I reach My hand through to you, through all the debris of your egos, all the effluvia of a million generations of resistance and depravity. Yes, I use this word purposefully, and now I will explain.

My beloved, precious, beautiful ones, as I give this gift to you I have one thing I ask in return. As your fingers touch these pages and your heart verifies for you their truth, *please give your life to Me, and then promise with heart and soul and all your being not to take it back. Draw close to Me and allow Me to be personal. And most importantly, that in every single thing you do with your SoulMate or toward the reunion with your SoulMate, let it be done in My Presence and in My Name.* In every single LoveMaking, say aloud My Name (in whatever 'gender' you choose to perceive Me). ALWAYS. Without fail, ever.

Now let Me explain this request. Let Me explain the title of this message (A Warning). We are, in working with LoveMaking, truly "playing with fire." Literally. With the fire of human feelings and with the power of human sexuality. This, of course, should be obvious. If absolutely every part of Creation came forth out of My sexuality, the union of Divine Masculine and Feminine, and you are My progeny – well, dear ones, this speaks for itself. Is the rest not obvious as well?

Beloved ones, this power and this gift that I am giving you in the early reunion with your SoulMate could go either way if you are not completely and carefully dedicated. Oh, I have asked you to guard your energy. I have explained how such things can be used unawares. Dear ones, human sexuality is powerful. It is coveted by those who would seek to derail your awakening. So while you must never focus on this, I must take this one message to explain it to you, graphically enough that you will not be careless, not ever, with this gift that I have given you. Shall I begin?

Unbridled lust is the exact opposite of Sacred Sexuality. See that you NEVER get them mixed up. For lust is the word I now use to describe what I will call "lower" sexuality. *"Lower" sexuality is sexuality that is disconnected from the heart.* Such sexuality has waylaid the progress of huge segments of the human population. Such sexuality is the reverse of Love. It is totally focused on the little self and it is completely connected to the astral realm, the "beltway of lost souls" that surrounds the Earth.

Here is some of the graphic part. This astral belt is dark and the beings there are still completely focused on fulfilling the lust they were consumed with in the body. So any time an embodied human begins to experience lustful feelings, hundreds (even thousands!) of these beings rush to that person. Getting ever more excited, they crowd around, each one trying to experience sex through this incarnated person. Of course they all want some of the experience, so every one of them is amplifying the lustful thoughts or feelings. So the person in the body may easily be driven to do more and more to satisfy the craving of those around him or her.

Then as the person on Earth begins the sexual experience, of course their partner becomes a "feeding station" for these astral entities, too. This couple's thoughts, actions and energies become even lower vibrationally as their passion overcomes them. *Now here is the worst, dear ones. When this "reversed lovemaking" or lustful exchange reaches a certain pitch, a vortex, or tunnel, opens into the astral realm at the vibrational level they are operating on, and they become the embodiment of the anti-Christ. Please pause to think about this.*

If you are becoming ever more fully the embodiment of Love, then it must make sense to you that the reverse is true, also. That the whole "reverse pyramid" of beings who are what we are calling the forces of anti-Love will also need people in embodiment in order to be fully present in the world.

I do not like being graphic and creating these images and feelings in your minds and hearts, but, beloved ones, it is worth it. Why is it worth it? I now ask every single one of you to begin a continual prayer with two parts. As you continually experience the grace and upliftments of your journey through Sacred Sexuality, through the creation of Love, *I ask that a portion of the Love you create always be used to protect and bless all who come in contact with this information. I ask you to pray to Me to be a continual part of your LoveMaking.* Of course, any prayers you can offer for the people trapped in the astral level will also be of great benefit.

There is every difference between what is normally called passion and what we are evolving into in the union of SoulMates. Thus, I am trusting you with a powerhouse of energy when I offer this information to the world. *I am trusting that true Love will be your goal. I am trusting that the energy of these messages will keep them flowing to the right hands and right hearts. And they will.* But here is why I am giving this message. There are many of you who have both types of sexual desire within you. This is what I must address. *For what has been considered "normal" in human sexuality cannot serve as your standard.* Please listen. It has been considered normal for human beings to engage in "fantasy" while having sex. I am not naming this LoveMaking yet, so you can see I am making a distinction between sex, as practiced in the world, and LoveMaking, as practiced in the heavens.

Fantasy cannot be considered normal for Sacred Sexuality. (I did tell you I would be graphic. For, of course, I know everything that goes on in the name of lovemaking – without capitalization!) You cannot be with your partner and be anywhere else in any part of your being. Especially your mind.

Now much of what is done in worldly "lovemaking" is based on dealing with the results of the horrible abuse and misuse of human sexuality. Oh, beloved ones, My heart cries out to you. Come back, beloved ones. Come back to My loving arms, My tender encircling of your beings, and let My soft warming light heal all that has been done to you. Oh, precious humanity, you were never meant to be hurt like this! But I can tell you that *only My Love, embodied as your SoulMate, can heal you.*

As to the gruesome details, a huge number of human beings, especially women, but certainly men also, use or experience very distorted tools for arousal. Most of these are the symbolic re-enactment of some abuse, coming to the surface again and again hoping to be healed. This is what most of the deviant sexuality truly is. My Love can heal it. My Love will heal it. Through your SoulMate. But the only way My Love and their Love can do so is for you to rise up to meet us. Open the cells of your body – for it is in the cells that every bit of the abuse and the hurt is recorded. *But do not allow the replaying of the lower sexuality behavior that has been your sexuality until now.*

Dear ones, if you are reading this and it does not apply to you, rejoice! Rejoice with heartfelt prayers of gratitude. Rejoice with every precious cell of your body and every atom of your larger being. *Pour your compassionate Love on those to whom I am speaking. For they are in the millions.* And they are many of the beings of light.

It is time to heal it all through the beautiful golden healing power of Love. As you open your bodies, as you open your cells, much will come out to be transformed. It is imperative that you keep yourself completely focused on the light, focused on higher Love. It is imperative, dear ones, that I am a part of your LoveMaking. Trust Me. Trust Me to be present simply as the shimmering light of the truest Holy Union. The Holy Union of two beings whose Love will heal everything it touches, including every part of both of them. Trust Me to lift you in a beautiful cocoon of light, oh, beautiful butterflies of the spirit that you are. Fledgling creators. Cells of My very heart. As long as I am present, you can know you are protected. Whatever is released from you, whatever patterns you have held in mind and body, will gently float up to Me, to be transformed into pure Love, into Christ Light.

Do not indulge, dear ones, in any old ideas or feelings about sexuality – but notice them. Notice them and give them carefully to Me.

If I had My preference, of course, I would not ever even mention this. But sexuality is SO powerful and I am allowing you to enter the Holy of Holies out of natural order. *Normally your vibration would be perfect "Love Without Ceasing" before you would draw your SoulMate.* So there would never be any possibility of anything emerging between you but the glorious union of Christ. *But to open the great heart that is humanity, and to open it on time, I give you access to your SoulMate before you are perfected.* This is my dispensation to you which I shall discuss later. In return, I ask for your diligence. I ask those of you who are firmly with your SoulMate in sacred union to will the safety of our beloved humanity again, again and again. I ask each one of you who choose to have your greatest Love to carefully dedicate your heart and soul to Me.

Beloved ones, keep your eye on the prize. My sweet humanity, I know how shadow-filled this world can be, how confusing. So I will do My part. I will reach through to you, individually and in these messages and I will help you find your way as you lift your bodies and your sexuality from the swamp of powerlessness created purposefully by those who serve anti-Love. I will show you, precious ones, how to have orgasms of the heart, where what begins in the limited areas of your body now allowed to be sexual can be moved by your Will into sweeping waves of Love.

Be present. Be present in the moment with your partner, in full consciousness. Hand Me any embarrassment, any pain, any pulls to fantasy or "acting out" of such. Just "toss it upward" through that channel created by your union. Then keep coming back to giving Love, not only from your heart, but from every cell of your body. Completely open yourself.

Be sure to say My name (a prayer in the beginning might be easiest). Then just keep giving, for the *difference between the forces of anti-Love or anti-Christ and the forces of Love, of Christ, is easy. The first is always focused on getting; the second is always focused on giving.*

Makes it easy, doesn't it? For if you are giving, in any situation, anyone who might want to use you for lower purposes would not be able to, for in the law of attraction, getting and giving are complete opposites.

Getting was necessary for awhile as you built an individual identity. You had to figure out which things belonged to you, or belonged with you, but now we move beyond this. You move into the higher energy streams, which are ever and always pouring forth in giving. Join in, dear ones! Join in! Give everything you are to your SoulMates – even for a minute - and you will understand. You will at last feel right. Your energy will be flowing once again, for getting is a stagnant thing. You may obtain but you are not refreshed. Giving, of course, opens your being to receive. Giving then pulls into you that very vibration at which you give.

Dear ones, your power has been taken from you carefully by the simple idea that one must GET something in relationship. Especially in sexual union. I know the power that has been lost to you. I'm trusting you to reclaim it, for when you do, its power will illuminate the world and bringing you home will be easy.

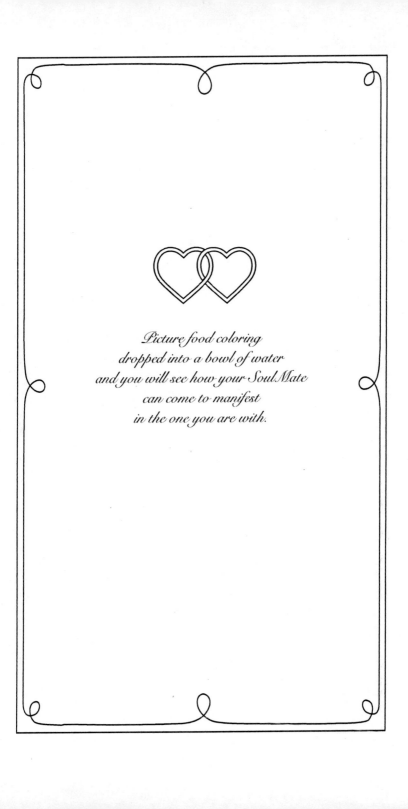

Picture food coloring
dropped into a bowl of water
and you will see how your SoulMate
can come to manifest
in the one you are with.

Clearing the Passageway for
the Flow of Love
And Thawing the Ego of
Your SoulMate

Beloved ones, I need you each to be the Hollow Reed, through which I am pouring Love into humanity. Being this open connection, you will begin to see just how much Love we can begin generating — generating by your Will consciously multiplying all that I send through you. Can you even imagine this? Who could possibly pour forth more Love than I? You would think that nothing can. But that is not true. Together, we can move into a completely new level of Love's reality. *In you I am multiplied.* Remember this. For you are those pieces of My heart. Within you I am expanded. I am multiplied. You are meant to surprise Me, to take what I am and to make something new of it. Can you see how this would be so exciting to Me?

Here is how this process begins. As you open your heart, My Love begins to be drawn forth through you, starting something that could be compared to a siphon. The more you pour forth Love, the more of My Love is pulled through you. However, in order not to taint this flow of Love coming through, you must "clear the channel" by removing your ego and any personal Will. It is at this point that you must come to understand that you must relinquish your Will. You must give yourself completely to Me and ask that only My Will be done in and through you. When you make this commitment and you raise your vibrations as you reach for Mine, it is a time for great rejoicing.

This giving of your Will clears the passageway into and through you completely, for there is nothing left to block the way. Thus I am free to pour through your being the full measure of My Love as the Living Waters of Creation. This flow becomes a river of light, a great cascading waterfall of Love that is a real and powerful substance as it rushes through your being. It is a force that can and will accomplish anything when directed by consciousness. The best image for your mind right now is that of a waterwheel, of the kind that is used to power a gristmill. The water's power turns the wheel that grinds the grain to feed the people. The Love now pouring through you is a very real substance that can be used to produce or accomplish anything you wish. You can use this power, the power of Love surging through the channel of your being, to produce all that you want and need directly. All you must do is place what you want (the idea, the desire, and the concrete plan) in the mold and fill it full with the substance of Love.

Now even of yourselves, as you become these clear and beautiful channels of My Love pouring through, you can accomplish these things. However, there is currently some interference. At this point, you are living in a world that is still very dense. What this means is that the molecules of energy here are moving very slowly, thus creating something very solid. As I have explained to you, beloved ones, Love in its natural state is *hot*. (This should make you smile, for certainly this applies well to your sexuality, and you will shortly see how perfectly.) Now, living here, no matter how much you reach for Me and lift yourselves up, it is very difficult to get beyond the slow heaviness of matter or the density of things that are moving so slowly.

So on your own, even if you open to Me, clear out your channel by giving over your Will and asking Me to do My Will through you, by the time the substance of Love makes it all the way through you to this current level of density it is very hard to mold anything. It is difficult to shape this Love into anything useful and very, very difficult to mold it into anything and send it forth from you. More than likely, it would not sit there before you if you were even able to shape the Love into something before it congealed.

The answer to this, of course, is your SoulMate. It is the passionate exchange of Love in a definitely heated state (a cosmic, loving "smile"). Sacred Sexuality. Then, dear ones, as your great Love together lights the fires between you, this glorious exchange of divine LoveMaking keeps the substance of Love in its molten, flowing state. So the first thing that happens is that all of My Love that I continually send through you and to you remains usable. Even in the great density of life here on Earth, in this slowest of all physicalities. So the Love that I pour through your hearts and your being, the Love that pours forth through every possible particle of your physical being has the possibility of spreading, of going forth to heal and love, to warm, and thus unfreeze, the world.

This in itself is the most amazing gift. *In a very short time, in an ever-widening circle, the world around a SoulMate couple becomes less dense. Why? Because the substance of all Creation is Love. And this Love is heated by the warmth of your passionate generation of the dancing, flowing heat of true LoveMaking, and the actual density of the physical substance around you is raised up.* This occurs because of the warming effect; and because like attracts like, and higher vibration always is more powerful. So the movement of Love in and around you will speed up the substance of which everything is made that is touched by your Love. All of this can also be multiplied exponentially by your consciousness because being made in My image and likeness, you are a creative force, especially when united in the balancing Love of the SoulMate relationship.

Thus you can together take the Love pouring through you, warm it up, amp it up, speed it up in your Sacred Sexual LoveMaking, and then you can create with it. Not only can you send forth the Love itself, but by your conscious agreement, you can multiply it. Then, once multiplied, you can send it forth. You can direct it, create with it; bless, open and unfreeze with it. Then, as you do this, you enter into the law of Giving, which is My Will that all that you give forth will return to you multiplied. Not just measure for measure. More than this!

We have spoken of all of this before, but dear ones, I am presenting this to you again. And I will again. And again. And again. Because it must become as familiar as your own name. As familiar as the feeling of the heart of your SoulMate. As familiar as the body you are currently wearing. And there is another subject.

As you experience this union of Love with your SoulMate, it is your purpose to bless in every direction — to pour forth the Love and the effects of its presence. Above and below, within and without.

Now, let me speak about the cells of your body, even of the atoms, and the energy of Love that keeps the electrons in their orbit. These, too, are living solar systems. Certainly you remember that in your science classes, as you saw the electrons moving about the center of the atom, many of you thought that it resembled a solar system. It is. I realize this may not fit with your current mental programming, but were you not so programmed, it would make obvious and perfect sense. You are the Logos, the God, the two of you together, who pour forth the great rays of Divine Masculine and Divine Feminine that bring order to your inner universe.

You are responsible for the upliftment and spiritual (as well as physical) well-being of these inner universes. You can listen to them as I listen to you. I ask you to gently allow this into your consciousness.

I realize this may be quite a stretch for some of you, yet easily accepted by others. As you awaken together it will happen automatically that suddenly you will begin to have knowledge floating up into your consciousness from this inner universe. You will also understand how nourishing the Within, as well as the Without, is going to be very important to you. For this is a tiny peek at your multi-dimensionality. So far, what looking you have been able to accomplish has always been upward and outward. This is certainly fine. However, I am introducing you to the expansion of your consciousness. You need put no other attention on this now. Just allow it to live softly within you. In its own time, as your Love deepens, your consciousness will easily be able to accommodate it.

Since I am offering quite a controversial message, I will continue on. I might as well open you to every possibility. Whatever you cannot relate to currently will at least be in your consciousness – a seed planted awaiting that warmth of spring.

I have asked each of you to put forth the call asking for your SoulMate, with the intention that your SoulMate manifest in your life by pouring Love into the one you are with. If you are not with someone, then I have asked you to draw, attract him or her into your life. Here is what I wish you to do while you are waiting.

First, you must remember the density with which you are currently encumbered. Then, please remember that it takes the heat of moving Love to melt this physical world. So *if you are with someone who is not yet manifesting the recognizable vibrational signature of your SoulMate, I ask that you begin on the higher, less dense level and work your*

219

way down, sending the melting qualities of moving Love to thaw your partner and thus allow the dancing, joy-filled essence of your SoulMate entry!

How you will do this is, first, open your heart. Become the clear, ego-free channel of My Love. Call for My Will to be done in and through you, and *remember that it is My Will that you be united with your SoulMate and that absolutely nothing is higher priority.*

Now place yourself in union with your partner. Sexual union, please. While making Love, ask to be shown how far down into density Love is able to flow between you. You will get this in a number of ways. You may see it represented in your bodies. "Can't even get into the head." "Through the head and down to the throat," and so on. Or you may see a column of light stretching above you to Me. These, of course, are symbolic representations of a vibrational reality, but this is what you need.

Then, once you have some sort of understanding of the energy flow, the possibility (or lack thereof) for the substance of Love to flow all the way into your relationship, I ask you to begin to work on this. *Use the energy of your Love as it flows from your heart to thaw the channel, the column, the opening between you, to warm, to heat the molecules of your bodies and your consciousness and heart so Love can make it all the way through both of you.* Especially use the energy of your orgasms to rocket upward and wake up your beings.

I can promise you this will be effective, for you are bypassing the ego. You need say nothing about what you are doing if you don't want to. You need not worry about violating another person's Will because you are reaching for their higher Will – the Will that is beyond the ego's little will, and the higher Will is always the reunification of SoulMates.

This I can promise you, for I have created you this way. It is only the little will of the self-centered ego that would ever resist Love. This should be obvious to you. Yet as the higher Will and your sacred union with the higher levels of your SoulMate warm the cells and the substance of your partner's being, eventually even the ego will be thawed and the truth of Love will make it through.

Dear ones, it is only when this happens that you can really make any significant impact on the upliftment of humanity. The channel of your SoulMate beings must be cleared from the highest part of your inner divinity (known to some as the I Am Presence) down into and through your human hearts and into the world. This is very important. *Love can only come into the world in fullness by those who are embodied here.* In other words, it is only by your Free Will that divine Love can take up residence in you, and through you to humanity and the Earth. *So your goal is to contact your SoulMate on the higher levels in their higher Will and to work Love down from the most ethereal to the most physical and then out, to bring Love into the hearts of humanity.* Of course once this flow is happening, then you can refer to the first part of this message and begin assisting the flow and generating even more Love as my beloved co-creators.

So the message I have for you is do not wait for the ego. Do not look at your partner and see the recalcitrant ego standing in stone-faced resistance to Love and give up. Please do not ever give up. Do not think that surely I must not have told the truth when I said that your SoulMate will come to you through the one you are with. The ego will be the last part of your partner to unfreeze. But I can tell you that even while that ego remains in clench-fisted resistance, you can have a miraculous experience of making Love with the higher part of their being.

221

You can make Love with your SoulMate and know it, experience it and, temporarily, your partner's ego may not even feel it. *But they will.* This I can promise, because the warmth of real Love is irresistible. Love is the highest substance in Creation. It supercedes everything else. So once real Love has been brought into active motion by you, sooner or later the ego's barriers must melt. Love always takes priority. That is a fact. Call it a law of Creation. For I am the greatest truth of Love. Actually, I am All That Is. So in My presence, all else must recede.

Isn't this exciting? *Dear ones, there is a revolution of Love happening in the world like the thawing of an ice age. The frozen glaciers of lower energy, of darkness, of belief in limitation, are being melted, being superceded.* Every one of you can use this knowledge to open the frozen places, in yourselves and those you Love, until the truth of Love is fully present.

One last thing: for those of you who are not yet with someone, the process is much the same. By opening completely to My Will in you and as you, you connect to the flow of Love. Then *you will direct it to your SoulMate in perfect trust of their presence with you.* For in truth, they are with you. They cannot be anywhere else. Remember this. You are two halves of one cell.

Then the same thing will happen. You will attune your SoulMate to your Love on every level and by the law of attraction, bring him or her to you. Since the physical is the slowest and densest, you will most likely have the experience of his or her presence on higher levels for a time before the physical self is drawn to you. But don't worry. It won't be difficult having patience because you will be with your SoulMate on every level that becomes unfrozen. So your experience will increase as your Love and Mine thaw the ice of the density of physically manifested reality. Then you'll recognize each other here, in third dimensional reality. Immediately. There will be no doubt, no questions about the validity of your feelings. You will know him or her, because you've been together.

As you can see, I am pouring Love forth in ever-greater quantities. *This is the Decade of the SoulMate. Please, call yours.* And please help spread the word. It is time for the melting of the limited lives of humanity quickly into a molten river of Love that will heal the Earth and everything else it touches.

If you are in doubt, check with your own heart. Go beyond your own ego. The proof is there. This I promise you.

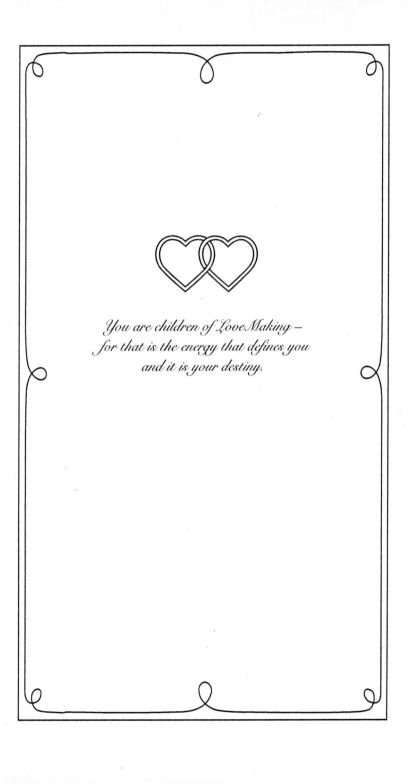

You are children of LoveMaking –
for that is the energy that defines you
and it is your destiny.

Awakening the Body, Opening the Cells and Preparing for the Union

I am here, as always. When I come close – meaning when you reach for Me with heart and soul – you can feel the upliftment. You can see the gentle golden light. You can feel it, as it sings within you, as it vibrates with a definite energy.

It is this same energy that is speaking to your cells, dear ones, when you Make Love with your SoulMate. For truly, there is a raising up of light as your energies are heated with Love. Then they begin a dialogue in which, in the unspoken language of Love, your very bodies greet each other. Your atoms reach for each other. Hungry for the food of life, of light, they too are merged in a sexual communion of such grace that through it you can become Ascended Beings whose home is light, who become the examples for humanity of the union of SoulMate Love. In this union the very atoms of your cells change. The electrons within them expand their course – into the "figure 8" of infinity, into your union as one being.

I want to speak to you of your bodies – of the truth of these vehicles, of the destiny of Love that awaits you. I want to say to you that your bodies have an understanding of unity, of Love, action, power and union that can bring you out of the trap of the illusion. Your bodies exist in a simplicity of life in which the way is easy. It is the simplicity of grace, which is the acceptance of the miracle.

Oh, beloved ones, your bodies are a miracle of Love. Can you picture them? Can you see how incredible it is that your consciousness has gathered unto itself all that you need to experience your life here, in this physical world? Now I come to whisper to you an even greater truth. Within you live communities. These communities of intelligences have been drawn together by the law of attraction. They are given life by you, and this life that is contained in your bodies is sexual energy. It is the energy of Creation. My energy.

You have learned to reach outward and upward. Yet to love perfectly is to experience this moment as the doorway to your SoulMate reunion, to ecstasy, and thus to co-creation. It is time, then, to begin to communicate by going within.

Dear ones, your bodies are sleeping. The cells, the atoms, are essentially holding still. Yes, I know, physiologically things are happening within you. But *on an energy level almost all of you are frozen, or moving very slowly. It is the heating up, the waking up of your beloved bodies that is the step up to becoming the New Man and the New Woman.* It is simply the awakening into higher, faster, lighter vibration that is the spiritualization of your bodies. It is the increase of light, or more correctly the transmutation of your bodies, that brings you into what is named the ascension, and the clearest, fastest way to accomplish this is the reunion with your SoulMate, especially on the atomic level.

How then do you love each other free? *How do you open up the spaces between your cells that you may see the background of eternity in the openings between them?* That is what we are doing here, in this powerful LoveMaking that is Sacred Sexuality. *And how do you join every part of your entire physical existence in the exact pattern of Creation,* thus opening the lock that has kept this a separate reality?

Oh, My beloved ones, you do this by loving each other so fully with such passion and giving that your very atoms reach beyond you to your Love. Since thought creates the pattern, you must choose this, and since feeling creates the substance, you must throw ego, caution, fear, reservation and every belief in limitation away! Then you must call Me and, heart and soul, I ask you to pray for this joining that is your destiny, and you will begin.

You will begin with the tender goal of waking every cell in your beloved SoulMate's body. Consciously. Having awakened the cells, you will open even more until you are both revealed to each other, truly, in every atom of your being. There, dearest ones, you are standing at the Altar of Creation. You will have in your hands as you touch your SoulMate's body, the very forces of Creation. Yours for good, or for ill.

Choose the good. Choose the complete union beyond any and all ego, and you will truly call forth those electrons I mentioned and your beings will be knit together in a pattern of energy that is so powerful that it is the equivalent of the atom bomb. Only now you will grow into using it to heat your homes, to traverse the world, to free all the beings of the Earth, My humanity, and the devas, nature spirits, and energies of Creation. **It all begins with the gentle, loving, passionate touch, in reverence and devotion, as you lay your hand in greatest Love upon the body of your SoulMate.**

If your heart is open, which it will be if you have connected with your SoulMate (on whatever level you are currently working), when you place your hand upon the body of your SoulMate, that Love pours out through your fingertips. Do not press upon their body because that would actually stop the flow. Then, holding the thought that you are giving yourself completely in Love, feel your Love pouring through your fingers.

Dear ones, sexual arousal is the ecstasy of the body if it is fully connected to the heart. Sexual arousal is your body getting ready for the SoulMate. It is your body moving

227

the energy of Love into every cell, opening it as a flower opens in the sun, allowing the bees to pollinate it. So are your very cells opening to receive the atomic energy when the full union takes place. Please listen and feel this with your intention. Just as a woman's body heats up in LoveMaking in preparation to receive the man, so too does every cell in a woman's body, once heated by Love, open up in preparation to receive the electrons from the man into the actual cells themselves, thus becoming impregnated with the new life – the joined human being. (I am using man and woman for convenience, but this refers to the inner charge, of course, not the genitalia.)

Speaking of genitalia, in these oh, so dense physical bodies, it is only the most overtly sexual cells/organs that have remained "alive" with energy flowing, and then in a limited way. Or worse than limited. If the heart is not engaged, beloved ones, these energies actually become reversed (a triangle pointing down) and thus draw only the energy of the anti-Christ.

Every cell in your entire body is sexual. Every single one. Now this will require some shifts in your thinking. The only reason that orgasm at this point in human evolution only involves (or mostly involves) the genitalia is because those are the only cells/organs that you believe are sexual. You have no idea how limiting this is. Not only how limiting in terms of your potential but also how limiting in terms of your experience. So just for a moment, please use your imagination and picture how it would feel if every cell in your entire body experienced not only the full glorious waves of exaltation that is normally focused in your sexual organs, but even more. Imagine an absolute and complete exaltation of being in which you are essentially poured into your SoulMate – merged – consumed in a holy union that literally blazes forth to fire you, to turn the "metal" of your normal being into the "gold" of your awakened and joined selves.

Now picture your hand reaching forth to touch your beloved SoulMate's body, and in that touch, it communicates everything you want to convey about how much you love him or her. Everything about all the glorious gifts of Love you want to pour upon him/her. About the wonder and beauty of the amazing body they are expressing. In that touch is every possible intensity of focus and intent of your burning desire to greet and to nourish every single cell and to reach within the cells unto the atoms. Unto the very seat of Creation where Love has now come to dwell on Earth. Unto the Christ Child. For that is who your beloved is. And that is who you are. And it is in acknowledging this that it is brought to life.

So you run your hands upon the body of your beloved SoulMate, as they also touch you in the same most holy and sacred way. It will be sexual. Remember. Remember what you are doing. Remember that you are waking the cells into their capacity to be sexual beings, connected to life, ready, ultimately, to be rejoined in the sacred union of transformation. This takes tremendous giving, dear ones. There can be no ego. As the energy becomes focused in the traditional way, focused in the overtly sexual areas of the body, *spread it out*. Take that very energy, dearest ones, and use it to heat the rest of the cells to wake them up. Use it to unfreeze them! Is this not perfect? That you can do this? Keep allowing the sexual energy to build, keep spreading it through the entirety of your body (this part you must do yourself because your partner does not know what you are experiencing).

I have already mentioned to you, but will tell you again, that this is the point at which, together, you are generating Love. Out of all of Creation within Me, you can create new Love by your Will, your intention. So at this point in LoveMaking, this is what you are doing. You can send forth this Love to thaw or heat up humanity as well. You can deliver new Love into the world. And you can, in the sacred space created between you, manifest whatever you choose to create.

This is an amazing gift, and to learn of it is awe-inspiring and can be very powerful. But I must encourage you not to focus exclusively here (or even very much). Why? You are too "young in the Spirit" to know truly what to create. It is absolutely critical exactly how you build your creations (you do not want to draw the opposite). And you will far better serve humanity by fully learning to embody your Christed union, for such will draw to you, unfailingly, all the amazing good that resonates with this perfect force of Creation you are now embodying.

That is the point. It is for you to embody the Christ of God, My living son and daughter. This done, the entirety of humankind will be enlightened by you.

We will, of course, explore this deeply-needed information and the powerful truth of the SoulMate alchemy. What I want you to see here is that it is now time for this door. *Sacred Sexuality and SoulMate Reunion is the path to the awakening for which you are waiting. I want you to understand that it is right here, available right within the things that are part of this physical plane existence.* Yet through this reunion of SoulMates, everything is changed, including these very bodies through which you are expressing. Through your Love they will become bodies of light. They will then simply *BE* the vehicle of your ascension, your awakening with ease into the real truth of your being.

It begins with the perfect trust to completely give yourself to Love. It proceeds through the miracle of completely conscious loving touch and the conscious directing of sexual energy until every single cell is singing in the glory of your union.

Thus will I lead you, My beloveds, step by precious step, touch by magical touch, until the sacred mystery of the communion of the living Christ is fulfilled – as you become the transformed substance. You become divine Love.

I will speak to you honestly and openly. Any embarrassment is part of the lie of disempowerment that has served to rob you of your most powerful energy, that of your sexuality.

Two last things will conclude this message. As you are learning this process of awakening, spend the majority of your time consciously using the sexual energy generated to wake your cells, but do spend some time giving forth the Love you are generating as a blessing. Be sure to choose to experience this extended arousal as ecstasy (or as close to ecstasy as you can get it). Do not allow it to become uncomfortable in any way that you are maintaining this arousal and not moving toward orgasm.

However, for as long as you desire after you have spent absolutely as long as possible in this aroused state generating Love, then proceed to orgasm together completely consciously. Use the orgasm to unify your bodies. Picture its energy shooting you upward together as your energies are braided together in ecstatic union. You can, alternately (though not as often), use the space created between you (the SoulMate Womb) to create what you want or need together. Hold it clearly in your minds in that space and energize it with the energy of the orgasm.

Secondly, if you do not believe you are with your SoulMate, **do this anyway**. Make Love with your partner in this holy way and trust Me, for I have explained that beginning to make these choices will begin to move your SoulMate to you. In miraculous ways. For this is the SoulMate time of the world. Reach out in reverent touch.

Hold this vision of your SoulMate in your mind, and watch for changes. Do not let a little thing like your SoulMate's currently lacking physicality stop you at all.

If you are not with anyone, then do this in your imagination. See it and feel it. Picture your LoveMaking and how it will be. You may envision appealing physical features or leave him/her fairly nebulous. The important thing is the open heart and the feeling.

You are standing right on the line with one foot in the New World, another foot in the Old. Please energize only the New. You will draw it right in to you. Dear ones, love your bodies. So very few of you do. Yet they really are simply congealed light, moving too slowly to function as they are meant. All it takes is the great softening power of Love to bring them back to perfection. But dearest ones, it cannot happen without your Love.

Heaven is going to be
the whirlwind of indescribable ecstasy
in which you paint the glory of your beings
across all Creation
as you are joined in holy LoveMaking
with your SoulMate.
Heaven is stars and worlds,
galaxies and a kaleidoscope of life
pouring forth before you,
as your joined hearts are illuminated
by your consciousness
and given substance by your Love.
This, dear ones, is Sacred Sexuality.

The Ecstasy of Our Cells

Oh, My beautiful ones, I wash you in the greatest Love that humankind has ever known, a Love that is unshakable, true, glorious, meaningful. Most perfectly this Love is shown to you in the Love of your SoulMate. In the joy and the ecstasy, the tenderness and protection, and passion and explosion of light that occurs when you touch.

Let Me lead you to another awareness. Loving yourself will bring you to your SoulMate. Loving yourself will reveal your SoulMate's presence. Remember how deeply and perfectly your SoulMate is part of you? Dear ones, if you can look truly into your face and hold the greatest Love and truest tenderness, you will suddenly begin to get glimpses of another face right beside yours, another set of eyes whose joy you will find reflecting back to you.

Many of you do not have true Love for yourselves because you have not understood your own depth. You haven't understood the majesty of your being and the substance from which you are made. But if you know, dearest ones, when you are looking at yourself that you are looking at your SoulMate, it really will change how you perceive everything.

When you look at your hands, I want you to picture the hands of your SoulMate's perfection. Picture those hands that you never tire of watching, those eyes whose depth reveal the truth of the greatest universes. See the heart that holds all of My Love within your being, radiating from within your chest like a tunnel, traveling endlessly within and endlessly without.

You must always see yourselves together, you and your SoulMate. So I ask you to make a promise to open your heart to yourself as you open to your SoulMate. As you do so you will begin to make the shift. There will be an exchange of Love that is that very rhythm of life. You will grasp the resonance, a resonance between you and your SoulMate that comes from acknowledgment of the great Love you share.

It is a resonance of Love, Love that you are giving and Love you are receiving at all points between you. You are giving yourself Love and you are giving your SoulMate Love. It is Love you are receiving from yourself, and Love you are receiving from your SoulMate. As this energy, this Love, is exchanged between these points, it creates an opening through time and into the moment of the eternal Creation, the NOW explosion of My joy, My ecstasy of giving, the force behind Creation.

These things are well beyond the ability of the mortal mind, the mind that is in linear Time, to understand. It is this little mind that we must now transcend. Trust that your heart is now waking to understand the language of Love, the language of eternity.

Let me tell you *the key word and the experiential doorway: ecstasy.* My beloved ones, *the great moment of Creation is happening NOW.* All is pouring forth in an explosion of joy that has poured forth All That Is. It is the union of the two parts of My Being, the great SoulMates, the Divine Masculine and the Divine Feminine. Oh, it is the great and glorious union. It is the pure and glorious magnificence! *It is, in a grand and glorious sense, the Cosmic Orgasm — the climax of My passionate desire to give Love and the deep knowledge of My being as it accepts that Love.* (Remember that second part – as it accepts what is given.)

236

It is the ecstasy of the great union that is the ongoing momentum bringing all of Creation forth, NOW. Your mission (should you choose to accept it...a little cosmic humor) is to find the way through the hall of mirrors to the eternal NOW, thus connecting not only your life but all life in this manifestation to the real life energy. The moment you do, Earth can be saved because the truth will become stronger than the illusion with every single choice. Every success. Until at last the hall of mirrors will fall away. It will have too many holes in it!

The way you do this is by connecting to the ecstasy. The only way to truly connect with the great explosion is through the true connection with your SoulMate. Now before you begin asking things like, "What about those not with their SoulMate?" I will answer you. *You who are not yet consciously in connection with your SoulMate must fully accept and acknowledge the truth that your SoulMate is with you.* Dear ones, he or she has to be, whether you can see them or not. I have explained this to you earlier. *So if you do not see your SoulMate in front of you, you must love yourself in his or her place and trust that right in front of you, behind that reflection of your face, your eyes, your hair, your mouth, your heart, is your SoulMate.* It is truly like looking through a two-way mirror, only you are on the reflective side. All you see are your own eyes, even though your SoulMate is right there, on the other side.

So as you pour your Love into your own eyes, it will get through. It will go right through the mirror and - ZAP – make connection. In that moment where pure Love is flowing, you are in the NOW moment. For that moment, you switch background and foreground. You are jolted out of the illusion and suddenly you catch a glimpse of the truth beyond the mirror. You are lifted up in complete and pure ecstasy. You are in communion with your SoulMate. You are in the world of Love.

How long you can continue the experience will be determined by how long you can remain free of attachments, free of thoughts, free to experience the NOW — as you reach across the divide between the worlds.

Even if you do have your SoulMate in your life with you, you may still use this technique of connection. Why? Because it is still unusual for a couple to be able to truly connect purely at this level. It is rare to have the attention and the control to open both beings at once in the presence of the other. Thus, even when you have drawn your SoulMate and recognized them as such, you can still very beneficially practice the choice for ecstasy through loving yourself. As you do love yourself, you are raising all parts of you – body, mind and spirit – as you use different ones as the doorway. This is wonderful.

To take this one step further, please realize that **the atomic truth, the NOW experience of each cell of your body, is completely and very powerfully connected to the great explosion of Creation.** For if you remember, the cells in your body are, at present, the most pristine enactment of the dynamic of Creation. The inner life of each cell is the cosmos, in Creation. In orgasm. In the exploding NOW.

Dear ones, if you allow this truth to fully manifest within your bodies, your bodies will simply explode into light. This is what you are calling the Ascension, or spiritualization of the body – raising it up. This is exactly that process, alive, in action, in the cells. Thus to experience this communion that will allow you to be raised up as Jesus was raised up (and many others) is simply and purely to allow the truth of your cellular being to manifest. Right now it is prevented, absolutely, by the decisions of the human mind and Will, creating the consensual reality here on Earth.

You have read many accounts of beloved spiritual masters making their Ascension as they sat in nature and had a realization of the beauty of all things. These accounts do not speak of the SoulMate. But I promise you their SoulMate was there and was experienced in that moment. For what often happens is a person sees such beauty, experiences such ecstasy of life, that they are instantly connected to the ongoing ecstasy of their own cells. They then go all the way "in" and through to the truth of their SoulMate, because the moment they allow the experience of ecstasy in full measure, in that moment they are returned to the full reunion.

If there are disparities – if the new communion, the new choice for ecstasy does not bring connection – then you can be sure that beliefs got in the way. But even if those are present, the communion of the two into one *will* occur. It just will not quite make the shift. You can believe Me that the vibrational resonance is building, set into increasing motion.

The biggest thing for you to carry away with you is the knowledge of choice for ecstasy. Oh, dear ones, in every moment you can have it. You must have it. And it will light up your life. And every single time when the lightning strikes again – when you are enlightened – your SoulMate will be revealed to you ever more clearly.

SoulMates are returning into manifested reality, every level, every moment. Each decision to experience ecstasy, to live in joy, to acknowledge the truth of Love's blossoming, Love's grand explosion, is to align yourselves with the truth of Love and SoulMates.

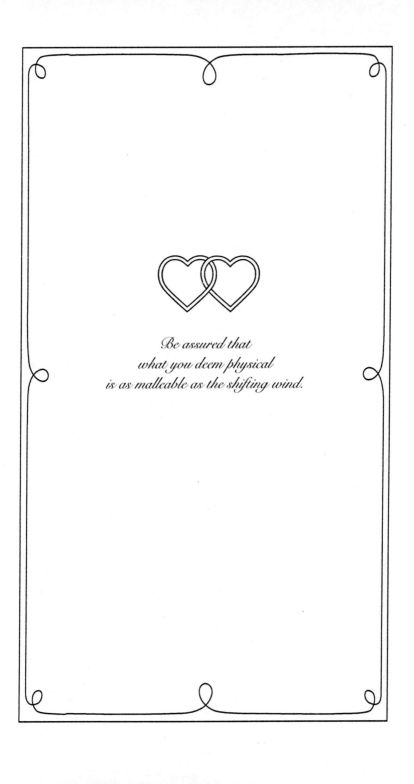

Be assured that
what you deem physical
is as malleable as the shifting wind.

Training Your Feeling Body
for Ecstasy

My precious ones, I will speak to you now, gently and supportively, about how to weave ecstasy into the most difficult moments! The *most* difficult. For all of you who are dedicated to the blazing forth of light, it is these moments – the most challenging – that hold the greatest opportunity.

First I want to remind you of a few important things.

Love is a substance.

Feeling is energy. (As you have heard – e-motion, energy in motion but I must remind you that we are speaking only of the energy/feeling of the heart and above.)

Thought is the mold. It is how you create the form for your creation.

How you actually create is to heat Love with your Feeling (heat/energy) and using your Will, pour it into the mold you've created with Thought.

Please do remember this. Here is what I want you to understand. In terms of actual creation and actual effect on your world and your life and on your beloved brothers and sisters, *feeling* is a critical ingredient, as well as completely choosing your thoughts so you do not create any loose thought forms to be filled with "passing" energy.

Thus, not only do you need to carefully choose the thoughts that will create your reality, but to actually *bring alive* the creation you must have dynamic feelings. Oh, best of the best – you must have ecstasy. So this is yet another reason why LoveMaking, the most sacred SoulMate union, is so powerful. Not only do you create while you are Making Love. Though I will keep teaching you how to deeply bless and dramatically change our entire Creation while LoveMaking, *I also ask that you carry a regular supply of ecstasy.*

All of you, on every level at which you can share this glory of the SoulMate union, are generating a supply of energy that can be used to serve humanity in many ways. For, dearest ones, *the energy of ecstasy is the true fuel of Creation.* It is the truth of My being. It is not only a unifying consciousness of utter joy but it can be used to fuel everything in the world. You can ultimately run your lives with it. You can create heat and light by calling forth this energy and then directing it by thought.

ECSTASY is the highest form of energy in Creation. Ecstasy is your natural state. So in your natural state you will use this energy to easily create all that you need in every area of your life and world. And you will be in complete and total joy. In ecstasy, obviously. Thus your every moment will be easily lifted on wings of joy up over any and every slower vibration. As ecstasy pours from you (please listen!), it will change absolutely everything anywhere around you. The weather will change. People will blossom. Things on every level will be grown and nourished.

Ecstasy must be claimed. It is your birthright. It is your natural state. The two direct sources of reconnection to your divine nature, your inheritance of ecstasy, are your SoulMate and your direct connection to Me. With great joy I say to you — claim it ever more fully. *Dear ones, it is your feeling experience that is the power in your life.*

Some of you have understood this but you have not been able to hang on to the experience for a long period. This is the next big step. For you now understand the choice of heart over ego, and have made this choice an integral part of your life. *Now every bit as important as choice of the heart is the training of your feeling body. I mean the lifting of its vibration to the level of the heart and the enthronement of ecstasy as the absolute ruler of your internal kingdom.*

Dearests, you already know that every moment My light pours in purely upon you. You know that you qualify that energy by the vibrational level at which you experience it. Every single moment it is qualified, whether consciously or not, and of course, its qualification becomes your reality. If you allow it to fall into the lower vibrations, it becomes part of the illusion. It becomes a beam of light bouncing back and forth between the mirrors of the distorted consciousness, creating more of the reflections you already see.

Or, you can keep the vibrations high. You can keep the energy as ecstasy. Not only will your life be ecstatic; not only will you warm and thaw the beautiful being who is your SoulMate but — dear ones, this is exciting — the energy of ecstasy will reveal the perfect truth of everything it touches! Listen to this again. It will reveal the perfect truth of everything it touches!

This is why I have been showing you ecstasy, speaking of ecstasy, reaching through the clouds of "maya" to touch your hearts and lives. I tell you that feeling at its highest level is ecstasy. This is what you are to have with your SoulMate. *When you are carrying a "subdued" ecstasy every moment, you are hooked up to that beautiful vibration and thus you can be, at any moment, a conduit for ecstasy in the world.*

Oh I want you to grasp that this is your nature. I want you to understand the glory of a human being who has opened himself to this joy. I also ask you to realize *truly* that we can no longer afford, in any way, to allow the misqualified energy of the world to affect you. For if you are going to be your destiny, My LightWorkers, to warm and thaw all human hearts, oh, dear ones, you have to take charge of the energy!

So just as you are learning to uplift and make another choice when you feel the ego rising up, so must you always find the way to choose ecstasy. You always have at least two avenues. You can come right to Me. I can quickly and easily lift you up. Or you can go to your SoulMate. You can pour Love upon him. You can ask for the complete instant re-immersion in the ecstasy you have shared together in the past. It is *so* effective. And you can now see what we are building here. In the SoulMate relationships, every couple is given access to continual ecstasy through the experience together.

Ecstasy is the New World. Just as you must move beyond ego to heart, so you must move beyond all of the lower emotions in every form and nuance and into a pure experience of ecstasy. This done, you are qualifying the light that pours forth to humanity every moment as that of the New World.

I ask each of you to find ways to ecstasy. Find things that work for you and use them. This is, beloved ones, exercising your Will. It is exactly like choosing the heart over the ego. It must become a way of life. But, oh, all of you, there is yet no way to explain what an impact this will have. Please suffice it to say that this will be one of the most important parts of bringing the whole of humanity into self recognition.

When you are living ecstasy, you will automatically draw to you the out-picturing of your destiny, and you will be in ecstasy doing it. Since ecstasy is your natural state, you will effortlessly find yourselves seeing things as they really are. So while you can use ecstasy and thought to easily create, you will be in such perfect joy and Love that your greatest good, your very highest possibility, will be drawn into your life. Moment by moment by golden moment, you will be in alignment with My greatest truth of you.

Feeling is the energy that powers the creative forces. True feeling is the energy that will unfreeze the world. Every moment of it will be glorious ecstasy. You, together with your SoulMate, will be a force for Good/God simply through your presence. I will teach you more every time you touch your SoulMate and every time you reach out for Me.

Remember each of you is an "energy sorter." As it comes in, *My light is drawn first to those with the vibrations that match this light most closely. This means that you of high vibration have the opportunity to qualify everything that comes in.* Please listen. This means that, can you sustain it, you can "place" every bit of energy coming to humanity. And then, even more — you can send it forth to heal and bless every single human being, as well as Nature and our beloved world.

If you miss your chance, the energy settles to the next level where it is qualified by the 'normal' human consciousness. This, of course, keeps the Old World in place.

Keep your feelings UP. Thoughts are step one. Feelings are step two. And they are more important. It does not suffice to simply be "serene and non-feeling" with thoughts centered on Me. You must generate or choose ecstasy as your energy (or emotional) reality. *So, you cannot simply open the heart. The feelings of Love and ecstasy must become your home.*

245

I will assist, as will the SoulMate relationship. For when you open to either, you will be in ecstasy.

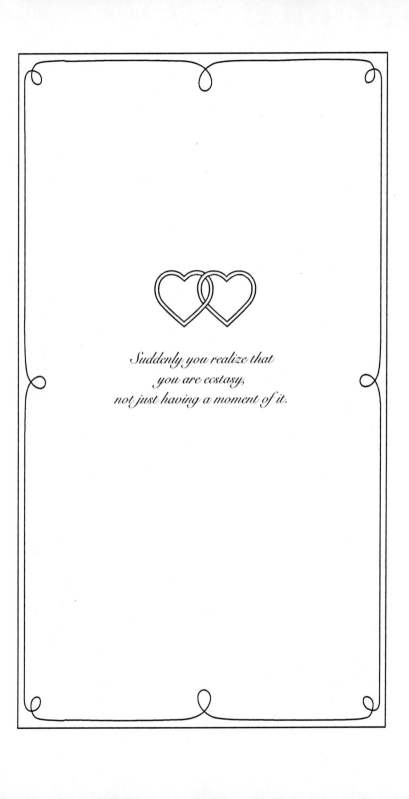

Suddenly you realize that
you are ecstasy,
not just having a moment of it.

Complete Communion
with the Ecstasy of
the Ongoing Moment of Creation

I speak to you again about ecstasy, one of the most important subjects we will ever discuss, and in discussing this, I am addressing every nuance of sexuality and of LoveMaking. I must because it IS the most important experience available to you. So, you must now "get over" any embarrassment or hesitance in *opening up the heart and soul of the gift of being human: LoveMaking.*

Sacred Sexuality is the key to human awakening for this age. It is HUGE, as you would say. Consequently I say to everyone whose eyes rest upon these words that any resistance you have felt while we have been exploring this topic, either intellectually or with your SoulMate, is absolutely the work of what you would term the "dark forces." Dear ones, those who have wished to keep ego enthroned in the world have worked diligently to degrade and pervert the most holy of all human relationships, because if you, My creation, believed that sex was sinful, it would create the psychological travesty that you see in the world today. *Sex is linked in human minds with everything and almost anything other than divinity.*

Sexuality is meant to live in the midst, the middle, the apex, the crown of a human relationship. It is to be the doorway to the Christing of humanity. I will tell you why and in a personal way — not in great cosmic terms. *It IS a reflection of the ongoing Now of Creation. It is the experience that is the glorious union of My giving forth and of the great ocean of My Love.*

I will explain to you *the bridge* that will now take you from the current world of limitation to the glorious union as Love with the ongoing Moment of My Creation of All That Is. That bridge is *ECSTASY*. Dearest ones, take a moment to open to this word. Open your heart and open your mind. Allow Me to touch you with My Love. Can you feel it? If you can truly open to the "touch of God's Love," My beloved ones, My touch is ecstasy. This is what I will always bring you. This is the true nature of My being.

When people speak of the Ascension, do you know of what they are speaking? They are speaking of *the complete consummation of someone's entire being in ecstasy.* Oh, yes! Let Me tell you. I will use My blessed, beloved Jesus as the example for he is most familiar to the most people, though there are many who have experienced this. In his worship of Me, as he opened his being, he began to feel My Love. First it was felt in his mind which became filled with prayers, with the complete breathless rush of giving. He felt he could not even think quickly enough, he had so many blessings he wanted to send. He would beg Me to help him include more, to bless more, to expand and expand his capacity for blessing.

Then it was felt in his heart. For as these blessings poured forth from him, My Love was drawn into and through him. So he began to experience My Love moving through his heart. When it did, the very cells of His heart opened, like butterflies or flowers in the sun. The atoms of his heart, precious beings in their own right, became filled with the *experience of My Love*, as it permeated every one. "What is this joy"? Jesus cried out. Tears ran down his face *as the essence of his heart became My Love for him.* This became his ecstasy.

The pouring through his heart then touched every other cell and the atoms of his cells began to dance in the cosmic experience of ecstasy. As I have told you before, Jesus was here with his SoulMate. When his entire being became ecstasy, it ignited hers and between them they "went through the middle" and came into complete communion with the ecstasy of the ongoing Moment of Creation. They did not have a physical sexual experience for there was no necessity. They were united in the glorious communion of Love in which they together became My will.

Let me return to what ecstasy means. For a moment, let Me paint for you within your mind and heart what it means. *Ecstasy is the complete overflowing of joy. It is when there is so much Love and so many blessings and so much absolutely inexplicable joy that every atom of your being is awakened.* Please listen! When the atoms of your body and your larger being are awakened by your experience of the above, they join together in sacred union themselves. Then, the center of the atom, that same Sacred Womb you share with your SoulMate, becomes filled with ecstasy. *Ecstasy is My experience of existence. Love is what I am. Ecstasy is what I experience. Ecstasy, dear ones, is what I am in — continually.* As you remember I am completely engaged in the one moment of the explosion of My Love into All That Is. It is essentially the great orgasm of Creation. Since time does not exist, it is ever happening.

Beloved ones, when your atoms become filled with ecstasy, the center of every atom *is beyond time*, beyond form. It is existing *with Me* in the Moment of Creation. This is why I have explained that LoveMaking can be your way Home.

To be Christed, to accept your heritage as My Love is to become that ecstasy. It is to have so much of you in ecstasy that you make the switch from identifying with the parts of you that are existing as a human being to identifying completely with the parts of you in ecstasy. Once this shift is made, of course, everything is forever changed. For the atoms whose centers *are* the ecstasy are light. That is what light is. It is atoms whose center is *Me*, vibrating at the *highest* rate. The highest rate is that explosion of Love that is Creation.

So as you experience ecstasy, as more and more of your being becomes made out of "atoms whose center is already Home," the more Me you become, the more light you are and the less you are identified with the smaller version of yourself. By saying the more "Me" you become, I do not mean that you fade into Me or disappear but rather that your actual makeup is as Mine. As your atoms become *God-centered* (literally and figuratively), you become *My Ideal* _____(insert your name here). As a part of My own heart, I know you. I know who you are in perfection, together with your SoulMate, when you are expressing My Will for you as you would say, or *My Will AS you*, as I would say.

As you become ecstasy, then, of course, you begin to draw God-centered atoms to you in every area of your life. Everything around you becomes only the perfect expression of whatever it is, be this food, or friends, or nature, or material goods. Even more importantly, the light everywhere present becomes yours to use. It is from this place of ecstasy that you will be able to "precipitate" – that you will reach out your hand and say "gold" or "money" and your hand will be filled with it. The light, *the God-centered atoms cluster around ecstasy*, because that is their nature. Then from that place of overflowing Love and joy and blessings, you will show your desire and the atoms will rush to provide it for you.

So far I have been speaking mainly of the esoteric reality. I have shown you before how these atoms within you (and around you) become the vessels of light that you can then fill and direct to deliver your blessings. Now I am explaining what the mechanism is by which you can go deeply within and through your very atoms, come Home. *It is through the connection to the glorious magnificent ecstasy of My experience of Creation.*

I have spoken about the importance of filling your mind and heart and being with the continual unspoken prayers for blessing for others — how you must pour forth those blessings, in the secret chambers within you, unknown to anyone but you and Me. I explained that doing this, *by your will pouring forth such continual prayers, I would be drawn into you to uplift your prayers and to uplift you. Dear ones, as you continue to do this and you open yourselves to Me, more and more and more you will be lifted.* As I join you, as I honor your requests and bless those you pray for, the closer you get to Me, the more you will begin to experience ecstasy. This is Part I.

Part II is Lovemaking. Now first let Me say to you that you can do this either way, Part I or Part II. Any human being can create his or her inner atmosphere to be so full of radiant Love and so full of the passionate desire for the blessings of others that this inner experience will cause your SoulMate to appear and together you can make Love, open the doorway Home into Christ Consciousness and you will go through. Or you can join together directly and openly with your SoulMate and through LoveMaking experience such ecstasy that your very atoms begin Love Making too and together you will open the doorway Home (Christ Consciousness).

If possible, the very fastest route is to do both. *When you have filled your being with the experience of ecstasy, the very atoms of Creation will "obey" you!* Obey is not the perfect word for they will take great delight in gathering themselves into *anything* you desire. *So it is through the experience of ecstasy that all the things you desire will be yours.* It will be easy to walk into a room and light it up, because you will feel the dancing electrons in your own atoms, so you will know the atoms intimately. I know this sounds what you would call "far out," and yet, dear ones, this is the truth.

You will find it easy to create heat the same way. Food? No problem. You will simply "create the mold" with your mind and ask the atoms to comply. You table will be filled with food made from light, directly. You will have less and less use for money as you are able to bring forth other things, but should you want it, the same principle applies. You will be fellow travelers with the atoms that you speak to and it will be a simple and delightful process.

Now – when I speak to you of experiencing ecstasy, this is what I mean. It is not the *idea* of ecstasy. *It is not* (listen here) *even the experience of being filled with light.* Many of you are experiencing this, and of course, it is a good thing, but it is not ecstasy. It is not an idea I am speaking of. *It is a consuming experience of great magnitude. Now for many of you the most effective access to ecstasy, to the experience of it, is LoveMaking.* And while I do definitely ask you to use both diligently (the sending blessings and the LoveMaking), I will focus on the LoveMaking most because this is the road to access for the majority. *It is with deep Love and joy at its possibility that Sacred Sexuality and the SoulMates rejoining is the hope of humanity.* So I want you to focus on and fully experience Sacred Sexuality as your main gateway.

There are what could be called "higher emotions" and what could be considered "lower emotions." *Ecstasy is the CROWN of Creation.* It is Kether on the Tree of Life. It is the highest of the higher emotions. Some of you have had little glimpses of what I can deem the "lower edge" of ecstasy. Now it is time to "go for it." I ask that this "study of ecstasy" now become your top priority. For everything else will explain itself once you have experienced this.

We are dealing with the most powerful concepts in human experience here and we are attempting to describe, in language, something for which you do not yet have references. However, I want you all to remember that your understanding of this is built in. So as you bring this into your life, it will be absolutely familiar.

Of course I am asking all of you to quickly rise above the ego involvement with sexuality. Please know that any hesitancy about discussion of sexuality, any embarrassment is part of the bondage in which humankind has been held! If you understand this one thing, you will free yourselves from prison, and it will be possible for you to listen to Me! So you can see how powerful even the edges of this work are.

Dear ones, this material is coming to you on wings of light. Thus I ask that you read and re-read this information as you learn together with your SoulMate in LoveMaking so that your cells will be "switched on" by the energies herein.

My beloved children who are reading this material, as you can see, we are entering a powerful phase! And I promise you that there will always be another! You will not ever stop somewhere and "be done." Wouldn't that be sad? No! Instead the true spiritual path is from awakening to awakening forever – for you are the extension of My Love!

This fact of the natural
"heat" or movement of Love is why
LoveMaking is the
most expedient and accessible way
to create Love!
At this level of vibration
(your normal world),
sexual arousal with
conscious connection to Love
is the only way to generate
real molten or liquid or flowing Love.
It reaches "up" vibrationally,
and makes the substance of Love truly available
in this dense physical world.
When you consciously maintain
this state of arousal
with open and dedicated hearts,
you are literally "unfreezing" the world.
You are bringing back the flow of Love.

The Dance of the Atoms
And the Freeing of the Cells

Dearest ones, let Me pour the light of My Love into you that it may illuminate your very cells. Let Me teach you the language and the movement of the constellations of wonder that reside within you. Let Me show you how the sunshine of your consciousness will bring each cell to life. Let Me teach you how to nourish the inner galaxies and the systems of life that are within you so that you may begin to ignite your body and become the starry heavens yourselves. All that is within you becomes the map for all that is without, and knowing this journey, you can follow it Home. Knowing this journey, you can ascertain the perfect course. Most importantly, knowing your inner universe you can become the causal force within your being.

Beloved ones, this is a study as grand as the great outer heavens which you have mapped and charted and which has served you well, giving you information about yourselves. Just as with astrology, so too can you use the maps of the inner voyage on many levels. You can use them to release and to heal, to acknowledge and to love – or you can become confused by them. But the study must begin. Because it is the knowledge of your inner self in union with your SoulMate that is the map of the journey Home and the key to Mastery.

I want you to focus on your heart. Yes, turn your precious attention there and gently let it rest. *Acknowledge your heart as the organ that is the center of your physical life and as the stage upon which the drama of Love is enacted in your life.*

Do you know how you can feel Me? How, when you open up your consciousness, you can commune with My presence, feel the truth of My Love touching and lifting you? *You can feel a vibrational shift that acknowledges My nearness. This happens because you are allowing yourself to expand your consciousness, to experience what already is.* Once you have made this connection, once you have allowed this contact, you can know everything. I know it doesn't seem this way yet, but it is true. However, were you to completely open to everything I am and thus all the knowledge you also contain, your circuits could not withstand the intensity. The equivalent of a divine electricity would pour into you. So you are protected by the law of universal attraction. *Nothing can come to you that you do not already contain vibrationally.* As you keep opening, so will the flow increase, so will the voltage go up and up until you are an open conduit for the truth and My light to the fullest degree.

You are the cells within My heart. This you know. Now I ask that you turn your attention to your own heart. *The cells in your heart are in exact relationship to you as you are to Me. How you love Me is how each of those cells loves you.* The level of your consciousness is reflected perfectly, as well. I have explained to you previously, My beloved ones, that your moment of awakening will be accessed when together with your SoulMate you reconnect with the Moment of Creation. This is accessed through the cellular dance of Love in which your own heart is connected, heated back into ecstasy, joined in the grand communion of exhilarating perfection and locked back in place as the *newly conscious* cells in My heart.

These concepts are larger than your language can currently convey, but if you will allow this into you by trusting My Love, I will bring you carefully back into the explosion of Love that will make every moment of your life ecstasy. Bliss. The most amazing Love for and with your SoulMate will connect you throughout reality, so the current of life flows unimpeded through you. You will consciously bless the great cosmic circle from the subatomic particles (very subatomic) all the way to the actual inclusion of your Will into the Moment of Creation – the moment that is happening constantly.

As you begin to allow these unimpeded currents to flow through you, you will become a true force for change. *A SoulMate couple, a cell of My Heart, is a grand and glorious source of radiant power with which you will consciously bless, transform and create.* So let us take a look at the atomic power of Love for there is actually a doorway to awakening in the center of everyone.

Dearest ones, I understand that it may be difficult to grasp what I'm telling you. Please don't worry. I am introducing an energy here more than anything. As we build upon it, you will see how exciting it is. You will also see the actual atomic dance of blessings as you send them forth. I have told you to bless others without ceasing; to bless within the silence of our own deepest self; to pray and pray and pray without ceasing that My Love be pouring through you to others. You also understand that what you give forth blesses you as you give it and it returns to you multiplied. There are reasons for this. *There are laws of movement that when you send forth a blessing you are sending forth an atomic delivery. You are sending forth "a SoulMate couple" on the atomic level of reality.* As you come to understand this process I will show you how, once you have sent it forth, to connect the atoms all the way up the scale of Creation - from atomic to cosmic - thus delivering perfectly the voltage, the life force, the pure and glorious prana (though you have no concept yet of what prana can be).

Dear ones, once you understand this process, it will be very helpful to you, helpful to humanity. Once I explain it to you, it will become something pure, something clear and simple that will allow you to charge up your blessings so the highest level of light is pouring through you, and the greatest level of Love is your reality. Once you move to this experience of the atomic power, all the concepts can fade away.

I will start by telling you that the way that you will charge up the SoulMate Womb of the atoms moving through you (yes, you guessed it!) is by divine LoveMaking! By consciously filling your heart with the ecstasy and plugging in every circuit to the original Moment of Creation. This is done solely by intent. However, it will require a continual purification and upliftment of your Love together to allow the highest accomplishment.

Once you have charged up the atoms of your being, beloved ones, these charged atoms will literally be dancing through your being, sparkling through your aura, ready for use as you send them forth as a stream of blessings powered by your continual inner prayer.

Of course, these atoms filled with the "Big Bang" energy will raise you up together, will bless and heal the two of you, every possible level of your beings and every ray of your manifested lives. In other words, all dimensions, all past lives, all other people whose lives have touched yours, all will benefit.

I have revealed to all who listen that there will be a New World and part of this New World is because the actual building blocks of creation, the atoms, are changing. No longer will they contain the life force at the level they have held within until now. Through the human reconnection of SoulMates, the atoms become the vehicles of the dynamic, exhilarating and gloriously powerful explosion of created life. *Oh, Beloved Ones, what this means is you can't stand still! Not ever again! I am pushing the "liftoff" button. You are now being reconnected with the Moment of Creation.* This is a very big thing!

You are aware of the fact that currently there are a limited number of people who could possibly comprehend this. Yet I will explain, gently and rather generically, that there is a new energy coming in that will literally wake up their cells. And I will ask all of you to say "yes" to this, as well. "Yes" to Love. And "yes" to the new energy that will bring vibrant health, joy and the ability to love and to be creative as never before experienced by humanity. Not even in the ages past where civilizations existed that were clear and advanced. Not even in the Garden, for this is a different time. Then it was a "going forth" and now it is a Homecoming.

As your ego is transformed into your identity as SoulMates and the charging centers activate the atoms with the new energy, you will become passionately dedicated to pouring forth blessings. Having created in your LoveMaking a supply of charged up atoms, these will ever be delivered by your conscious Will. As you send forth your continual blessings, every one will have a bevy of "passengers" to be delivered to the object of your prayers.

As these atoms pour through both you and your SoulMate, you will attune your own beings to this new energy, lighting you up as the light of Christ becomes the definition of your beings.

So the atoms become enlightened. Then of course so do the cells of which they are a part. Now, listen, *as this happens, your very cells will be reconnected in a new way to their original blueprint. Dear ones, this means that each cell will be freed of "the illusion." Each cell will be alive and conscious of how it is meant to be, conscious of its perfection.* And, each cell will know its harmonious relationship to all other cells. Freed from the lie of separation, all cells will become regenerating, as they were meant. ***This, of course, marks the end of death as you currently experience it.***

This cellular consciousness will also mean many other wonderful things. As you can tune in to your cells, you will begin to experience Creation, all of it, how every one of those cells connects to all the others, and, how every cell knows Me. The awakening will then be upon you in the most magnificent way. There is what I will call a registry of stars, where the lights are all connected and connected on every level. Imagine this as best you can and even the imagining will feed you.

You do not need to understand all of this consciously, but you do need to have a sense of it – a sense of the magnitude, the amazing beauty and the glorious ecstasy as All That Is becomes fully and consciously reconnected. Ah, dear ones, there is a generosity of Love that is the foundation of All I Am. What does this mean to you? It means that whatever great good you can imagine, there is more. Whatever Love you can conceive of experiencing, you must multiply. Whatever joy you can begin to envision, it is far greater. This I ask you to remember. So that, especially in loving each other, you will pour forth more. Expand your possibilities. Expand them now.

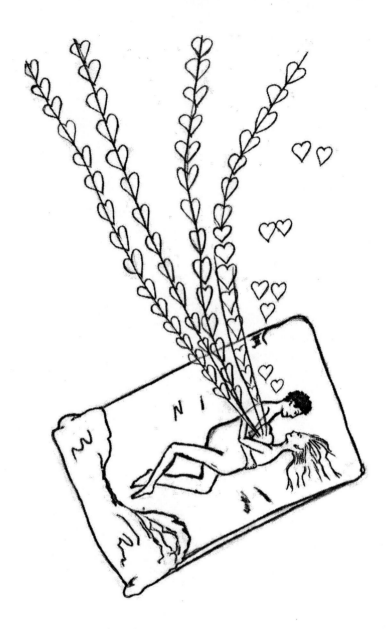

*Sending Love from the SoulMate Womb
to Unfreeze the Hearts of Humanity*

A Study of Light

The Cup of the Electron is Filled in the Sacred SoulMate Union

I continue to bring forth these gifts of awareness on every turn of the upward spiral, so your consciousness is ever expanding. Beloved ones, it never stops. The process of opening, awakening, growth, and understanding never stops for it is the nature of My being that I am ever growing and expanding. So relax with the idea that you can't get it all because you never will. There will always be another amazing discovery. There will ever be the treasure of new combinations and thus new life, new awareness, for I am always learning. That is the purpose for which I create.

So, knowing this, let Me softly pour into your eager minds something new. This is why there will always be the seeming repetition of what I have already given you, except that it will always have one shining new piece.

I will tell you about light. Perhaps we could say "Light 101," the kindergarten course (sent with a gentle smile). Yet Light 101 is a foundation course upon which all else will be built.

Light is essentially the energy released from the movement of Love. The movement of Love, especially in its true fluid state, puts off a flood of electrons. Each electron carries the actual brightness/light or heat equal to what was generated by the Love from whence it came. This heat is energy as you know it because it creates change. The electron delivers its heat to whatever it touches, but then the fact of the delivery cools the light, which then must be heated back up again.

The greatest movement of Love is the Moment of Creation. It is the LoveMaking of the two great elements of My being. So it is LoveMaking that charges up Love, the substance of My being and moves it. *It is, dear ones, LoveMaking that is the source of all life.* The energy released, the light is what keeps Love moving, keeps it alive, keeps it molten. It makes it able to generate its own light, which then pours forth to nourish other life. *It is the movement of Love and the energy generated therein that is life.*

The fastest moving Love creates, of course, the greatest light, for the energy pouring forth from such a union as Creation is beyond your current comprehension. However, let Me tell you two very important things about this light. First, it is embodied. Remember this? *I explained to you that absolutely every energy in Creation is held within a consciousness.* The embodiment of light is the electron. Because the electron is a conscious being, there is much for you to understand about being in relationship with electrons.

Perhaps most important of all is that since the electron is a conscious being, it is affected by other consciousnesses. In fact, *the electrons are meant to be a deliverer of energy. So they faithfully deliver whatever energy is given to them to deliver, by other conscious entities, for these beloved ones are intended to carry forth My light, to deliver it and then to be refilled and sent forth to deliver yet again.* And again and again and again. This is the circulation of life.

In a perfect situation, these electrons go forth, deliver this energy they carry to another life form, another design of Love (for Love is the substance of all Creation). Delivering the energy then energizes or heats up the Love from which that being is made, which generates more light. The electron then is refilled with this newly created energy and, having elevated the Love it found, it moves forth to make another delivery. This next delivery will do the same thing, only this time it will be the Love of the second being that created it. So as this new light goes forth, it draws more light into that being who created it. This process is what you have heard termed "qualifying life." *The quality of the energy/light that refills the electron either increases or decreases its original level of energy.* Thus light can and does become degraded as it moves into and out of other conscious life forms.

Every electron will continue on and on, delivering and being refilled forever. It will continually be raised up or lowered by the consciousness it comes in contact with. The only thing that can ever stop this flow is for a co-creative consciousness (like you!) to send it back to Me to be, essentially, regenerated. This brings it back into the very highest vibration. Vibration is the rate at which the energy is moving. Obviously as energy is released from Me at the moment of the ongoing explosion of My LoveMaking, it is moving. Very fast. Very, very, very fast. *So to send the electrons that come into your field of energy back to Me charges them way up and brings back the purity of their energy.* However, if they move into the energy field of you, then the energy they carry becomes your energy, right?

Obviously this is a way that you can lift and bless and bring the Love here back into a more molten state, especially through the union with your SoulMate. You can do an amazing transformation of this energy. You yourselves can refill it with that very energy of the ongoing Moment of Creation if you and your SoulMate reconnect to this, which is our goal.

Oh, dear ones, this is a rather technical message. It is so because this understanding will really serve you as we progress. However, the process I am speaking of here is the most magnificent. Oh, it is the cradle of Creation. It is the birth of the Christ Child as energy, through your LoveMaking with your SoulMate. It is the return to the Garden. It is the key to the direct route Home. It is the way that you, My awakened SoulMate couples, can instantly lift the world, accomplished by the reconnection of your Sacred LoveMaking with Mine (which you really are already).

When you heat up your Love, which is your essence, in conscious LoveMaking, you are sending forth a great fountain of electrons that are filled, or charged, with highest light, thus delivering the light of the Moment of Creation to those they touch. At first I have asked you to deliver this energy to yourselves. Why? To grow you quickly back to the ability to reconnect with the highest light, the ongoing NOW of Creation, so that even when you are not physically making Love you will be completely connected. Thus connected, there is an open channel through which these electrons can pour continually, not only when you are actually making Love.

One other thing. Remember how I have told you that Creation is ever growing, expanding, because that is My nature? It is because of My continual "orgasm," the glorious union of Divine Masculine and Divine Feminine that new electrons, new light/energy are always pouring forth, expanding the light, thus expanding All That Is.

Now I just spoke about your ability to "clean" and refill electrons, that they could come to you with lower energy and leave from you with higher energy – even the very highest. This will be something you will eventually move into together. I will continue to teach you, especially when you are together Making Love. Later you will be in such communion of ecstasy that you will be continually "joined" whether your bodies are engaged in LoveMaking or not.

First, you must wake the cells, for the cells are the communities that process the energy delivered by the electrons. So obviously they must be awake and on duty. *Dear ones, the Love here on Earth, in general, is moving so slowly that your cells have gone to sleep because they do not have anything much to do.* Your sexual organs and your own frequented "erogenous zones" are the only ones with much to do. Now obviously you are still alive. So energy must be moving through you. And it is. But, My beloved ones, *if this energy moving through you now is what I consider being asleep, what would it be like to be awake?* Think upon this!

So, as you awaken your cells, they become ready for ecstasy, because ecstasy is the feeling produced by the real movement of Love. *When you feel ecstasy, you can know that you have allowed into yourself enough light that your being is moving closer to your natural state.* You can feel how you are meant to feel, because feeling is the experience of the energy released from the movement of Love that is your being. The more fluid and faster moving your essence, the faster the energy, the higher the feeling, because the more you resemble your true nature. In such a state, of course, you will act only on Love.

So first you awaken the cells. You do this for each other best, but those not with your SoulMate physically can definitely still call forth their assistance on the higher levels and bring the energy into your own bodies. *After waking the cells, you will find that your sexual experience now encompasses your entire body.* Your sexual organs are not more or less sexual than any other part of your body. *Your LoveMaking becomes a complete and amazing full-body experience.*

Next you will begin to connect to the Moment of Creation. Your very atoms will be merged with those of your SoulMate. Your electrons will now travel in a figure 8 between you. The alchemical marriage will take place and you will be one heart, one being, one light. Suffice it to say that this figure 8 of electrons will open up your very atoms and allow connection with the NOW Moment of Creation ("the Big Bang").

At this point you begin running perfect light through the system, which is now the two of you as one. You are at this moment Christed beings. Not man using Christ energy, but rather you are the very Christ energy – the perfect electrons, pure, crystal clear. Your beings, the Love you are, begin moving at the rate of Creation. This is where you can change everything with a thought, a touch.

Yet way before you reach this point, you can create new Love as I do. For in truth the moment you intend this, it begins to happen. It is, of course, by our Will that this begins. The moment your heart is open you have access to All That I Am. The moment you join with your SoulMate, at least some of your atoms begin the figure 8 between you, opening the gateway to the Moment of Creation.

As this gateway is opened, dear ones, brand new electrons pop into your lifestream! You are then carrying within you at least some of the perfection of Love. These electrons deliver into your lifestream their cargo of pure energy, pure light, the highest light of Creation. Can you fathom this? The moment this happens you have begun the transformation. You are now carrying the Christ Light in you. Perhaps only a tiny bit, but it is **very** powerful.

Now many wonderful possibilities exist from this moment. You can amplify that light, consciously asking for its increase (a very good thing to do while and after making Love!). You can then refill that delivering electron and send it forth to transform someone else. You can send that electron back through the gateway to be refilled again and then you can accept the light into your being, or you can send it forth to bless another. No matter what, the delivery of even a tiny portion of this perfect light greatly uplifts the vibrational sum of your two lives as they become one.

The light received in SoulMate union is the perfect light. However, there is always light coming to you, essentially keeping Love alive, keeping even the most hardened individual with enough fluidity of substance that life may continue. This light comes to you in many ways. It comes directly from the beings that are your Sun. These beings in turn are continually receiving even higher or faster light from a greater Sun being. Light is also consciously poured to you by those beings who are the tender caretakers of humanity — those ascended ones who have walked your same human path and become one with the Christ Light, the energy of My Love, and also from the archangels and angels.

Light is also drawn to humanity from within humanity by LightWorkers like you, people who realize that everything is accomplished by Will and who then apply their Will to increasing the light in themselves and humanity. Those calling for light to be poured forth upon humanity will discover that such light will be always sent through them. So one is actually able to accomplish far greater things and still receive light themselves by doing this.

If one calls only for their own light, they will get it, but they could have accomplished the same AND lifted humanity for the same effort. Obviously this is the right thing to do — to give forth and be blessed in the giving. To add even more incentive for you, as well as the light coming through you, you will receive it again – for what you give forth always comes back to you. *This, then, gives you a glimpse of the upward evolution of Love. If you give forth, you receive far more in return, blessing you so you can give even more and thus be quickly raised up again.*

The only time I ask you not to focus on giving forth is when you are together with your SoulMate, awakening your cells, for to place your Will and attention there, on yourselves, will increase your ability to give forth more than a thousand fold easily.

I spoke earlier about qualifying energy, about sending forth the emptied electrons filled again. This happens automatically. The electrons go forth filled with your vibration of light (or lack thereof) unless you will it differently. This is how energy/life becomes misqualified. If your vibration at that moment is, say, fear, then fear is what will be carried forth. Now not only does this then deliver fear somewhere else, it draws more fear back to you.

This is why you must control your feelings. Feelings are energy. And how you do so, of course, is to control your thoughts, for thoughts direct your feelings, absolutely. So every single moment of your life these electrons pour into you, deliver to you life, and wait to pick up whatever energy you have to share. Now you can see why things are such a mess with humanity. *As the urgent call goes forth now for the readying of humanity, control of thought and feeling is the most important single thing a human being can do.*

Now you can consciously clean up burdened electrons. These are electrons that have held misqualified or negative energy and became caught in a downward spiral. Because of their cargo, they are naturally drawn to other lower vibration people and thus it continues. Such electrons would not normally be drawn to you unless you fall into negativity. But if you do fall into negativity, what an opportunity! You can then call to you and through you all those electrons drawn to you and carrying such energy and by your Will you can dissolve/transmute their cargo, refill them with Love, and of course, send them forth.

You can also choose to do this cleansing. You can, by your Will, bring lower vibration electrons in and cleanse them by raising them to your level of Love and sending them forth. This is what Jesus did and does in a very big way. This is what it means to "have your sins forgiven." Unfortunately, humanity does not yet understand that once one such as Jesus empties all of their electrons and fills them with light, then *they* have to keep them there. This is what he meant by, "Go forth and sin no more." But this "sin" as it has been called is energy. And what is energy on this plane? FEELINGS. So if someone goes to Jesus and is cleansed, it is his/her feelings that must "sin no more," or in other words, not dip into negativity. This, as you know, is not understood. So people wonder why even after "giving their life to Christ," they are still burdened. This is why.

Beloved ones, even before you are barely awake you are a fountain of light. The light just doesn't make it very far because there is no feeling energy and Will to push it (and of course there is not a great amount of flow).

This gives you much to think about. *Please think mostly about your continual decisions to feel ecstasy and Love, for if you do nothing else, these decisions will change everything.* Yet it is worthy of you to take these adventurous explorations of the mechanisms of Love and energy and consciousness, for it will ultimately assist you to hold fast to your decisions, because you will understand why, and this understanding will continue to grow.

The adventure continues!

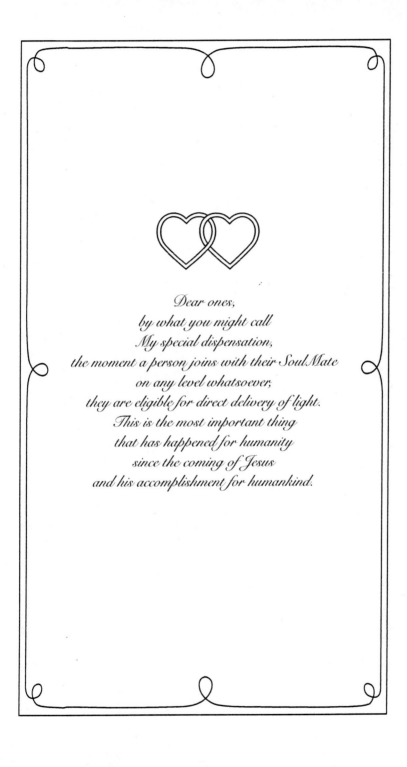

Dear ones,
by what you might call
My special dispensation,
the moment a person joins with their SoulMate
on any level whatsoever,
they are eligible for direct delivery of light.
This is the most important thing
that has happened for humanity
since the coming of Jesus
and his accomplishment for humankind.

My Delivery of Light
A Special Dispensation

I ask you to stretch forth to meet Me, to stretch your mind to encompass the vast and glorious truth of Love. Stretch open your hearts to allow the experience of greater Love than you have ever imagined. Allow My light to fire you to begin the process of illumination. *My beloved ones, you who are stretching to understand will be the light of the world.* When your very cells are illuminated by the joyous ecstasy of Love, you will become a living torch lighting the way for all the others. It is time, time for the illumination of Love.

In this stretching forth of your receptive minds, I ask you to imagine a greater light, the light of the energy released from the ongoing Moment of Creation. Imagine the light from the ecstatic, joyous, exuberant, exalted moment when I moved into action; when My desire to give, to share, to know all of My possibilities and have relationship became reality. Oh, it is here in the moment where the entirety of My Will to Give moved upon the Love that I Am, that the truth exists. The truth of ecstasy. The truth of giving. The truth of becoming one with your Will and Love in that moment where they meet. The truth of light. Beloved ones, light is the energy that pours forth from this glorious, ecstatic explosion of Love.

It will require every bit of your imagination, but please reach to touch this ongoing moment in the biggest way you can. Think of the most incredible LoveMaking you have every experienced, or the most glorious moment of pure ecstasy, and multiply it billions of times. Think as big as you can – of all the beautiful galaxies and all the worlds within them and ponder the very moment when absolutely every bit of it came forth. Now hold that thought. Hold that thought while I tell you that every bit of that entire experience is held within the light that is released. Released from the great joining of the Will and the Love of All That I Am.

Because everything in Creation is holographic, you can access this experience. It is yours. Dear ones, this access is the goal of your life, for you are experiencing this. You and your beloved SoulMate are in it. You are My heart! So if you just use a physical, human orgasm as an example (and a tiny one!), you are the part of Me that is most involved, flooded with all-consuming ecstasy; with joy beyond explaining; filled with movement like the beating of your human heart. You are pumping forth the essence of this Love and light to all the rest of My body! And what is all the rest of My body? It is all of Creation!

Are you getting a sense of how important you are? Are you feeling a glimmer of the magnificent communion of Love that you are? And remember – as above, so below. Not only are you the perfect Love that is My heart in action forever in the Eternal Now, but within you lies the very same intelligences that are the cells of your loving heart. So you can see at least a little glimpse of who you are. In this you can also see how urgently I call you back to the awareness of Creation.

Now that you have pictured in your greatest capacity the union of SoulMates that I Am, you can see also what the glorious truth of light is. *Light is the energy of ecstasy. It is the feeling of the Moment of Creation.* Please think a moment on this. The light that washes your world, animates your being, and fills and fuels the entirety of created life is the energy released from this glorious movement of Will and Love, which for your understanding at all I must explain as the One True Orgasm.

So the light that pours forth, streams forth, explodes forth, is the feeling of the Moment of Creation. It is being delivered to you. It is a gift, held in praise and thanksgiving by every conscious being of Love, for this is the very energy of life. The very energy of life. It is what animates and nourishes a creation that is so fantastic you truly can't imagine it in your current state. So you can see what this means: life is ecstasy!

Life is ecstasy. The very energy that fuels absolutely every living being, every moment for all eternity, the energy released by My movement, the movement of Love. Ecstasy. The energy carefully delivered to you regularly, without which you would cease to exist. Ecstasy. Held in reverence in the cup of the electron, it is brought to you, beloved ones.

Every single life form that has not forgotten its heritage bends its knees in praise continually for the miracle of light, for the miracle of light is the miracle of life. All who sing in praise of light, of life, find even more life pouring forth to them as their exaltation of life brings to them its own. (You remember that like attracts like.)

Dear ones, you have forgotten. You have forgotten the miracle that it is to be alive! And truly it is. For in this one moment, I understood the truth of giving. I understood that I could move, that My Will could move upon the waters of My being, that I had both Will and Love. So from this miraculous moment has come forth the ecstasy of life.

So I must now tell you that until you live in praise – in continual praise for the miracle – you will not be in right relationship to life. Until you can see the value of life in its perfect expression as light, the electrons cannot deliver their pure cargo to you, for your vibration does not match. You will, without knowing, push life away. Yes, you will stay alive. You will stay alive because foremost, that is My Will. So even the most "evil" human shall always have the same precious Will that I have. You are Me, after all, and you can receive the electrons filled with "qualified" light – those that carry a lower vibration that matches yours. But, it is time for you to have far more than this. It is time for you to have perfect life, to be perfect life, to experience perfect life, which is to accept in Love and praise the delivery of light that is ever being sent to you (though it rarely is able to deliver its bounty).

Dear ones, the plan is this. *When the light within you becomes as great as this glorious light I continually send to you, then the Circle of Life is complete.* You will then reclaim your full identity as the very cells of My ecstatic heart, at the Moment of Creation. Then every cell of your entire being will accept and receive perfect life. You cannot yet understand what this means. But I can tell you this. There are worlds within worlds within worlds within you, every one of which will then be free, free to live the ecstatic expression of giving life. The beautiful Earth is included in this, for She is an expression of your physical selves, the home you create around you, and all life upon and within Her will at last also be free to finally express the truth of who they are as life/light at last flows through them unimpeded.

This, beloved ones, is freedom. This is what it means to be Home in Me, to recognize life and honor it. Honoring it, giving it permission to accept the gifts of light that are continually being delivered to you – most often to be unconsciously refused.

When light pours forth in the Moment of Creation, it is the ecstasy of life. Pure and glorious. As it flies forth with the explosion of energy, the movement of the electrons sing in ecstasy. Oh, there is no way to explain this to you. But let Me tell you that just to hear it as it moves forth in purity would bring you immediately home to the truth of your identity. It is the joyous work of the angelic choirs to pick up this song and to carry it forth through all the dimensions, all the lands of Creation, and to make it available for all to experience. *Please ask for this.* As the light streams forth into denser and slower vibrational realities, it is harder to hear the song but it is there. Its melody is known in every particle of your being. Once again, any being hearing this song can do only one thing, burst forth in praise for the gift of life.

The electrons that carry this light, this life streaming forth from Creation, hold the charge of the receptacle, the cup, the carrier of life. This charge is feminine. Thus the Song of Creation is the most beautiful melody you can ever imagine sung in the lilting voices of the electrons as, pregnant with life, they go forth to bless. Oh, it will truly melt even the most hardened heart, the most "cooled" substance of Love. But, of course, the challenge ever is that it must find entrance, and only human Will can give it.

Oh, that you could see, could hear, could even barely comprehend these beautiful electrons streaming forth. How tenderly they hold their charge of life. How gracefully they swim through the cosmos, looking for any receptive life. In relation to humanity, these beautiful beings regularly fail to find but a few beings on Earth that can take delivery of this life directly. Those that find such a human are overcome with joy, and filled with magnificent gratitude, their new song flows quickly back up to Me, blessing profoundly everything it touches on the way.

Most of the time these electrons must deliver their light to an intermediary — to the archangels and to those humans already ascended. These beings then must step down the light, often way, way down, to deliver it to humanity. Thus, as you know, much of humanity is existing on a very tiny bit of life which, of course, translates into having very little light to see by and little life to live by. So the majority remain cut off because they do not have the Will or knowledge to raise their vibrations and to open their hearts to receive light, to have life.

Here, is the exciting part. *By what you might call My special dispensation, the moment a person joins with their SoulMate on any level whatsoever, they are eligible for direct delivery of light.* Dear ones, if you do not understand the magnitude of the above sentence then I will tell you. *This is the most important thing that has happened for humanity since the coming of Jesus and his accomplishment for humankind.*

There are others who have ascended and who also serve humanity in glorious ways, but Jesus also came with a similar special dispensation: that those who accepted and then lived by his message, would, essentially, be on the "fast track" Home. And while it may not seem so, I can tell you that had Jesus not come and had his message not been so widely accepted, even in limited form (remember this!), humanity would definitely not now have the above opportunity.

Take a moment, My precious ones, to allow this message to penetrate. If you call for your SoulMate, if you say "yes" to Love and open the door of your heart (this is a requirement, for without this you cannot make contact with any of this), your SoulMate will begin to come toward you. This I promise you. Then the moment you connect, whether or not you are together physically yet, you become eligible for the direct delivery of pure light. This will change your lives "in a hurry," as you say.

This dispensation is the only way that I could open you up quickly enough to accomplish your awakening in our agreed upon time frame. Since the reunion of every human SoulMate couple is a part of the homecoming, it made sense to use the one consistent heart message still accessible in the majority of humans: the remembrance of your SoulMate's Love. For as I have said, the survival of this encodement in your cells, which essentially tells you that you are missing their other half, is what fuels you to continue to reach for relationship. The survival of this memory of your SoulMate, with whom you fit "hand in glove" is what has kept you from finding the right relationship. Why? Because you *know* from deep within what Love should be like, and no amount of psychology or experience can change this knowing.

Now, dear ones, it is time for your longing to be satisfied. This search you have been on all your life for your mate, will bring you far more than you imagined, for it will bring you back to life. Nonetheless, there will be those who will have difficulty hearing this. There will be many who, although the "still small voice" keeps urging them, have become cynical. They have made the decision to give up on Love, and the one thing that it takes to draw the SoulMate is an open heart. So the work of those of you who understand this process is to find any way you can to help your brothers and sisters make the new decision and say "yes" to Love.

All of you have a SoulMate who is now accessible to you at the level of the heart. The most important decision you can now make is the decision to call him or her into your life. You do this by believing in their reality and by opening your heart, by making the call with true, dedicated *feeling.* Be sure that I am in your call, and be sure you have accomplished the true desire.

There are many of you who say, "But I have been calling my SoulMate and he/she has not appeared." Beloved ones, I must gently tell you that vibration is an unshakable law. Your SoulMate is a part of you, but you cannot see him or her or draw them to you until you have an open heart. An open heart creates a vibration of Love that is specific. Scientific. Unfailing. ***So if you have been calling and your***

SoulMate has not appeared, I must gently say to you, with much Love, your heart is not really open. You have something in the way. Something that is keeping your vibration below the heart level. It most likely is fear. It often is rooted in the past, in decisions you made earlier (in this life or others) that are keeping you from choosing Love truly, with open heart.

So if this is how you feel, that you have called to no avail, then I must call you to a deep self-honesty and a true and rigorous search for the earlier decisions or experiences or habits of thought or body or whatever it is that is keeping your vibration down. Dear ones, you could be one inch from the heart level and it would not work, for it truly is scientific in the best use of that word. Vibration is an impartial registry of the sum of your inner truth.

The exciting part of this is the same. Because vibration is a truth and Love has a vibrational signature, once you reach that vibration nothing can keep Love from you. As surely as the sun rises and sets, as surely as you have life, so, too, do you have Love. That Love will be embodied as your SoulMate. You can count on this, but you may have to do some excavation work and some prayers asking for assistance if there is something blocking the way.

Then you are here, in loving communion with your SoulMate. You can look into their eyes and see Me. You can look into their heart and see yourself, and you can join together in reverent, sacred union. Listen! When you make Love with your beautiful SoulMate and you touch their body in total praise for life, each and every cell within that body recognizes itself as Love. (Pay attention!) When that recognition occurs, every cell will open and your loving adoration will then reach their very atoms. The atoms, too, will open, becoming like a butterfly freed at last from the cocoon. The beautiful electrons with their cargo of pure and glorious light will penetrate the atoms (no, penetrate is not the word. They gently "land" inside the atom), drawn by the positively-charged nucleus, and the very atoms of your body and being will transcend their limitation and become ecstasy. This union is what you could call orgasmic. From this explosion of Love the electrons now carrying your perfect light, are pushed, catapulted. They leap forth and trade places with those of your SoulMate. Thus are you ever reunited in what I will call the Sacred Alchemical Marriage. You will then ever be united with your SoulMate in ecstatic communion with My own bursting forth in the One Moment, ongoing forever, of Creation.

To accomplish this Sacred Marriage takes a devotion to Love and thus to your SoulMate, that is pure and absolutely clear and uninterrupted. *It is to become one with the glorious praise of Love that is the light.* It is to touch in perfect Love, to see in perfect Love, and to completely open every particle of your being to the giving of Love. When you become that stream of praise and giving and convey this through your holy, tender, loving touch, it will happen.

For some of you this will be a journey, for I am describing here a clarity and dedication unknown by any of you yet (any who are not already ascended beings). But for others it will simply be a memory. You will grasp it completely in the span of a moment and you will become pure unified Love in the ecstasy of life. Yet whether it happens quickly or slowly, dear ones, every step will be a wonder, a joy yet unheard of by humanity. It is this that I now call you to. That in praise and gratitude Myself, I may welcome the awakening of every cell in My Heart.

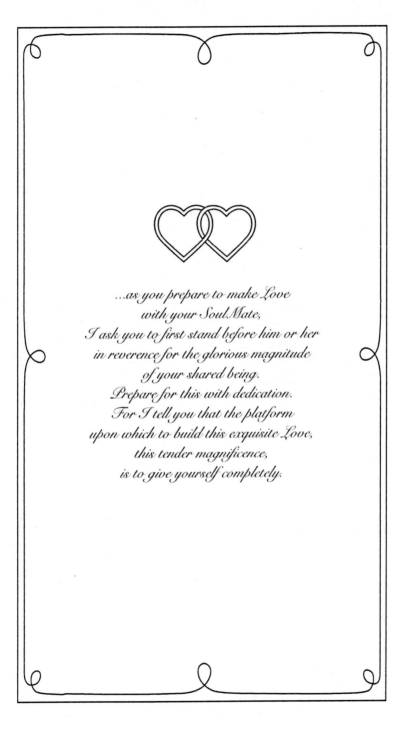

...as you prepare to make Love
with your SoulMate,
I ask you to first stand before him or her
in reverence for the glorious magnitude
of your shared being.
Prepare for this with dedication.
For I tell you that the platform
upon which to build this exquisite Love,
this tender magnificence,
is to give yourself completely.

Sacred Sexuality and Sacred Marriage

I ask each one of you who choose to have your greatest Love to carefully dedicate your heart and soul to Me, and thus we come to Sacred Marriage.

It is my desire that every couple conscious enough to read this book together choose to participate in a Sacred Marriage ceremony. You may already be married. This is another step. You may not want to be married in the "eyes of society." That matters not at all. It is My hope that you will want to be married in the Sacred Marriage that is meant to sanctify your relationship, to firmly establish Me at the apex of your union and to weave around the two of you a circle of light that will be fortified from that moment on by every being of light that is working with humanity.

What this marriage ceremony will do is amplify your intent consciously by sending it outward on the wings of Love to be picked up and augmented by every one of the angels, the archangels, the Masters of light, elder brothers and sisters of humanity, and by every one of the many beings who are here from other galaxies to help.

This ceremony, dear ones, is for you and Me. It is to lock into place your SoulMate union. And just as I mentioned, in any creation you must seal your creation in light to protect it as you bring it forth into manifestation. Thus will the Sacred Marriage become the hallmark of true marriage, the marriage of two light-filled beings with open hearts as they put forth their intention to fully manifest here on Earth as SoulMates.

It is this intention that will begin the sacred transformation, cell by cell, moment by beautiful moment, until the cosmic entirety of their unified wholeness is revealed and lived in physicality.

Oh, just to speak of this with you sets the whole heavens to singing! Can you hear it? Can you feel the great release of light that happens simply by turning your attention to your union with your SoulMate?

Sacred Marriage, done with highest intent and greatest Love, will create a channel of light through which you together will rise, protected from the astral level and any other interference. Do this, and then "weed the garden" of your mind. The light will be able to pour straight from Me. Then when you open your body, when even your very atoms unfold in trust of Love, you will be safe to heal. As the old hurts are released in the light, you will be held in perfection until this is what you become.

Oh, precious ones. Can you see this? Can you see yourselves together filling the sacred tube of light created by your marriage, filling it with the rising flame of your unified Love? First it will be a flicker. Then it will be ignited – ignited by your giving to your beloved. Then one will ignite the other and then back again as the receiver becomes the one who gives. Hearts giving, minds giving, cells giving, even atoms. The giving is the movement of Love, the ecstasy in which you have always lived in truth.

Then as the united flame of your Love reaches up, up, up, it calls forth the response. Singing in joy and praise and gratitude the sweet electrons come, released from My Moment of Creation as I looked upon your perfection. The circle is complete. You are back home, where you started, in the beautiful Moment of Creation. Yet having traveled the circle, you are One together in relation to Me.

At this moment all the energy of Creation is yours. You are the full embodiment of My Love. Christed beings, yes! But you have no idea what this means yet. Then the column of light that is your marriage vows opens, becomes a living fountain. Your living ecstasy, your perfect light of active, moving Love, pours forth to bless and bless and bless. It illuminates everything in all Creation, for you have taken My Love all the way down into this density and raised it back up, bringing this world with you.

It will work, precious ones. It will work. It is a daring plan, but I believe in you. And, I believe in the promise of those we call LightWorkers, that you will live to give this light to others, to lift and bless My precious humanity. Now you can see, beloved ones who serve the freeing of My frozen Love! Now you can see the powerful way this applies to you, for once you are united with your SoulMate, you will have the entire spectrum of light, the ecstasy of living, moving Love, with which to serve and bless humanity.

I can promise you, beloved ones, that My every hope is in this path of Love. Thus I have paved the way as best I can to give you every opportunity. Every opportunity to use your Will to do My Will, and every protection and blessing as you do.

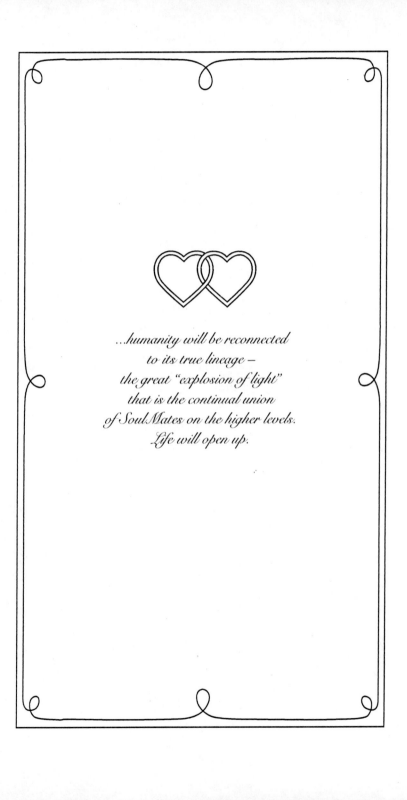

...humanity will be reconnected
to its true lineage –
the great "explosion of light"
that is the continual union
of Soul Mates on the higher levels.
Life will open up.

The Holy Communion
of Sacred Sexuality
Becoming One Heart

I speak to you now about LoveMaking. I am going to lift you up and show you the dazzling union of all Creation that occurs when two human beings, particularly SoulMates, Make Love.

I have explained to you the "story" of Creation — the great union that is the joining of Divine Masculine and Divine Feminine when those two parts of what I am are Making Love. They are every moment! The result of this is you, and this magnificent Creation, of which you understand only one particle, and of which you have experienced even less.

Yet I have given you the heritage of My Love. I have given to you this very experience. I have created you with the very same ability that I have. I have made you what I am. So you, My beloved ones, have the ability to join in the Moment of Creation.

Oh, you are My Love! You are My Love in every level of expression. You are activity engaged in the exaltation, the ecstasy of this great union of My being. But you have closed your eyes to most of it.

I have said to you often that you are My Love in form, yet in truth you are far more than this. *You are My Love in fluidic ecstasy of glorious cosmic union just as much as you are these limited physical expressions.* You have just forgotten where to look to remember this.

I have explained to you, beloved ones, how you are the expression of the Divine Masculine and Divine Feminine – for you could really be nothing else. You are the cells of My very heart which also contain every element of My being. Yet you are also these bodies, bodies that are filled with light. Your bodies are filled with the joyous celebration of every cell for the glorious gift of life. But, temporarily, you have forgotten this, too!

So here you are. You are listening. You have spent some midnights beneath the tutelage of the Moon as she spoke to you of the very tides within your bodies and their relationship to your larger being. You have heard the message of your own precious heart as the cells within it call to you just as you call to Me, praying for their Love, praying for the SoulMate.

Dear ones, there is no end to this glorious universe, this story of the explosion of Love that is happening now through all eternity. This joining in LoveMaking of the two parts of My being as the moment of My giving, My bursting forth, goes in absolutely every direction — from the ever expanding largest to the ever spiraling inward of the very smallest.

I do not ask or expect you to follow this completely at this moment. What I do want is your acknowledgment of the great majesty of all that you are, of all that you are a part of, and the great potential within it. *You are here in these beautiful expressions of Love you call bodies, the expression here in Time of the sacrament of LoveMaking that you are.*

To recognize this that you are requires the reunion of the two parts of your being. So, say that you are with him or you are with her. If this is on the level of the feeling body or the mental, this is fine. This is an acceptable place to begin, for those levels are completely real parts of your being —

closer to your natural fluid state, in fact. So if you begin this in your heart (feeling) and in your mind, I can promise you that the physical recognition has to follow. In other words, beloved ones, *I ask you to begin this experience now, on whatever level is most accessible to you.* If you are comfortable functioning in your higher vibration light body, that is even better.

This physical world is slowed, congealed, "hardened" to the point that you have lost your natural expression of graceful, dancing Love that is your birthright. Yet in truth these bodies you are using to express your totality are still not solid. Your bodies, dear ones, are only one small expression of you. It is like being in an elevator in a huge skyscraper, getting off on floor 13 and believing that floor is all of the building. This is what you are doing.

So even while this physical expression is truly, as you say, like "molasses in January," there is still inherent within it all the other expressions that are you. You can access every single one, every level. You can have every experience of your entirety of being by "riding the elevator of LoveMaking." You can go to any floor. You can experience the entire building. And the most glorious part is that you are ever in the loving embrace of your SoulMate and ever in the sweet upliftment of My Love as you do it.

Thus as you prepare to make Love with your SoulMate, I ask you to first stand before him or her in reverence for the glorious magnitude of your shared being. I ask you, beloved ones, to begin with the most important commitment to your relationship. Prepare for this with dedication. For I tell you that the platform upon which to build this exquisite Love, this tender magnificence, is to give yourself completely.

As you stand before your beloved, throw open your entire being, and as you do, so you will feel the hands of eternity come to place within you true power. For I remind you again that it is only in giving that you receive.

Many of you today are very concerned about being in relationship "without giving your power away." While this attitude has served a purpose in the balancing of the plus and minus energies in the mass consciousness, it becomes a great impediment as you step upon the true path of awakening. Dear ones, this kind of power is of the world, and here each moment is before you the spiritual choice.

All of those things that your beloved Jesus explained to you hold even truer today. "It is only by giving up your life that you save your life." This has been interpreted in many ways, but, what it means to you is that it is only by seeing your SoulMate as God and giving yourself completely that you will ever see yourself as God. *It is only by completely giving yourself to Love that the ego is released.* Please read this sentence again. Paste it on your wall. For in its simplicity is My greatest gift — that I have given you a real expression of the Love you are, in embodiment as your SoulMate. Can you grasp the great gift here? How much easier it is to give yourself to someone who stands before you, than to give yourself totally to yourself?

So your greatest act of empowerment is to completely give your power away — to place it before your SoulMate. This will grow you profoundly for in order to do this you must trust Love; you must trust your SoulMate; you must believe in My promises, and you must overcome your ego.

Having come in reverence and presented the "pearl of great price," your personal power, you are ready to begin. Now as you reach forth your hand to gently touch your SoulMate's body, you will begin a Holy Communion. In this communion you "eat and drink the body and blood of Christ."

Now before you bring forth any other references in your mind as to what this means, let Me tell you. *You, My beloved humanity, are to become the Christ in this age.* The Christ is the office of your spiritual awakening. It is the truth of My Love made manifest in the world. And just as Jesus, through his total communion with Love became My living Love, so too, will you. You too will become the singing ecstasy that is your birthright. As you become the Love of your SoulMate, you will know her body so deeply, in such communion, that your cells will literally be joined, symbolized as "eating the body of Christ." So too will your very blood become the song of One Heart that is the communion of your true SoulMate being. This I promise you. *This highest and most holy union of SoulMates in divine, tender, sweet, surrendered LoveMaking is the communion of this age.*

It is meant in exactly the same way as Jesus meant it, although few have understood. For when he said to those who saw him, "Take, eat. This is my body which I give to you for the remission of sins" (what he actually said was, "for the overcoming of the world"), he meant this same transformation. He meant that all who said "yes," who had this communion, would give themselves completely to him, just as you now give yourself to your SoulMate. In so doing, the same release of ego, the same raising up into Christ Consciousness occurred.

As you become the giving, as you release every single bit of your identity, as you reach forth to blend, to melt into him or her, as you give yourself to your SoulMate, you become the divine alchemy. In this communion of Love, which is the communion of Christ, the rushing blood — singing in your ears, responding to your fingertips — joins you together in one spiritual heartbeat. You will easily and automatically join your energy centers. As you do, dear ones, you become only the Hollow Reed, only the channel for My Love in your giving to each other. My Love is wrapped around you. Your hearts are joined, and a miracle of transformation begins.

The more you will that My Love be given to your SoulMate, the more open to My Love *you* become. The more Love you give to your SoulMate, the more Love is attracted to the two of you. Thus the more energy of this feeling of giving Love, oh, which is the very highest next to pure ecstasy itself, the more this Love heats you. You are ever more fluid. Your vibrations are raised up and up as your Love weaves back and forth, as each of you keep giving to each other until your very body opens up in ecstasy, and you become light.

In this moment you are Home. You are touching the truth of your being, and every cell is revealed to you as an exact replicate of your SoulMate union. In this moment you become a fully awakening fluid being on every single level of your being. No longer are you only on the "one floor" where you got off the elevator. Now you are experiencing every floor at once. Being here, in this state, at this point, then together you can use your Will and your attention, to experience any level of your reality and to bless that level, not only of your being but through your being.

Oh, and there is more. I understand that for some of you this is very esoteric. But as you begin to experience this communion and expansion of consciousness, it will become ever clearer to you. Right now we are using limited words to explain a "future" experience for which you have no reference. It is a little bit of a challenge.

In this glorious communion of Love, through the doorway of your unified being, you can do the works that

Jesus did (as he so clearly stated). Yet this is not the goal. It will, believe it or not, be incidental that by simply turning your attention and using your body at the correct level, you can heal and bless and raise up. *You will realize instead that granting this experience to every other human being will be the cry of your heart.*

You will understand through the blessed language of your body, both "heavenly" (raised up) and "earthly" (physical), how you are indeed reuniting (or re-zipping, as I have called it) every level of separation that came into being through your outward journey. Now you will be Home and all the illusion of separation will fade away.

Your very cells will be united – yours and your SoulMate's. I cannot explain this in terms you will currently understand. However, suffice it to say, this is the making of the New Universe. Your very atomic structure, once joined, becomes the foundation for a unified reality. I have explained to you that each atom is a universe at a different level of creation.

Do not worry about understanding with your intellect. Understand with your heart. Understand that as you lay your hand upon your SoulMate's body, you are waking the very universe of their being — the universe within as well as the universe without.

Now every cell and every atom of your bodies, as they merge, become the doorway also to ecstasy. Dear ones, please listen. As you heat up your atoms together with Love, allow the ecstasy to sing together throughout the beautiful joining of your being and you will begin to feel the pulse. At first you might believe you are experiencing your own heartbeat. But as you gently caress your beloved's body, as you hold yourselves together in the gloriously building sexual union – stay there. Do not go forth to physical orgasm. As you remain ever more sensitized, ever more swept together on the currents of divine ecstasy, you will feel it. As you keep giving and thus keep receiving the most perfect Love, your every cell will begin to pulsate.

At first you may perceive this as tingling. But if you continue to focus on the Now Moment, you will recognize it as the bursting forth of the waves of ecstasy through every single atom of your being. Ultimately you will expand beyond yourself in awareness. You will recognize your experience. You will know the greatest ecstasy, the truth of life, of Creation, of existence. You will be united with Me while remaining an aware "individual" consciousness. You will be united with the moment of Creation, the explosion of My Love into manifestation. You will experience yourselves as God — for you will experience all things as within you. You will be united with what you could call the cosmic orgasm. You will experience wave after wave of exploding ecstasy where what is within and what is without disappear. Rather than experiencing orgasm specifically in an area of our body, you will experience every single cell and particle of both of your bodies joined and extended to infinity.

There is no way to fully explain this in words, but in this moment you will be free. Foreground and background will certainly change. You will be cosmic beings, Divine Masculine and Divine Feminine. You will be in complete and magnificent communion with every single atom of Creation and from there you can choose! Because you are co-creators. Oh, dear ones, you can't fully appreciate this yet, but you will. You can experience it all and you can then choose what to do with it. Is this not the greatest gift? You can explode together into the glory of Creation and then you can come back. You can come back into illusion if you want, although you will never really forget. Or you can completely shift and become a guide for those opening after you. You can be here, in limited reality, or you can be there in the amazing wholeness of everything. But whatever you choose to do, you will have become an awakened SoulMate being for you will be One, not two.

So the recognition of Love and ecstasy, the heart and then The Unity (unified experience of All That Is as it is becoming) will be the experience. This may, however, take some "time" in your experience of things. Yet it all begins with one little step. Say "yes" to Love and call for your SoulMate. Then pay attention. For I will grow and stretch you until you can fit your SoulMate in the spacious Love and acceptance of your being. Then step-by-step I will lead you as you change your mind about what Love can be.

Those of you who have conquered fear will be the leaders. Only fear can stop your Love, stop it from bursting forth from you into your life. Truly, it is the time of the awakening to Love. And may I whisper to you that this new communion is what you are meant to experience. Ah, My beloved ones, *you are the church and within you lives the truth of every holy message that has ever come forth.*

What you think and feel creates what you experience, so choose to experience Love rather than the illusions of the ego.

♥ Choose to open your heart.

♥ Say "Yes!" Call your SoulMate to you. Be open as to how your SoulMate will appear.

♥ Pray with gratitude continually. This will get your energy (your feelings) up to the right vibration to…

♥ Begin to practice Sacred Sexuality. Invite the Holy Communion of your entire beings.

❤ Choose ecstasy. Love passionately by giving yourself completely.

❤ Travel gently or lead in complete faith into union with each other so fully you experience the Moment of Creation.

I am now placing your hand in the hand of your SoulMate; placing your heart as a treasure in his or her consciousness. Believe in miracles. I can tell you that where he or she was not one moment ago, they can be, fully present, in the next. Are you ready?

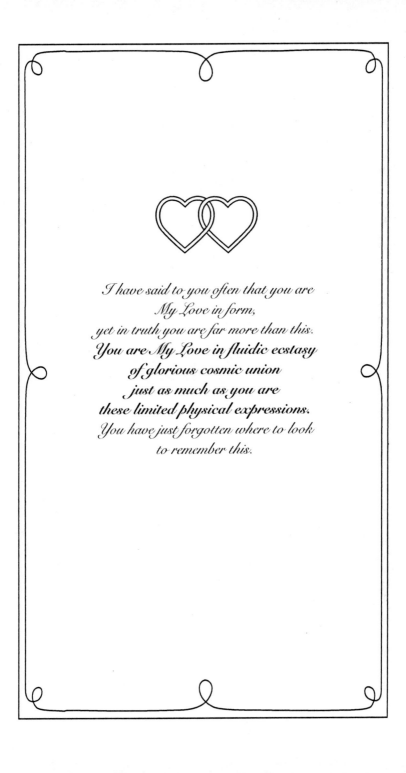

*I have said to you often that you are
My Love in form,
yet in truth you are far more than this.*
**You are My Love in fluidic ecstasy
of glorious cosmic union
just as much as you are
these limited physical expressions.**
*You have just forgotten where to look
to remember this.*

All of Creation is Passionately In Love

My beloved ones, raise your precious eyes to Me. Oh, it is the goal of this journey that you shall reclaim your life. I have taken you to the stars. I have brought you through the many levels of life's expression to the truth at the center of All That Is – the Eternal Moment of Creation. I have shown you angels – angels that hold galaxies in their care and angels as tiny as the electrons that carry you to the elixir of life. I have brought you to the sacred truth of your SoulMate. In all of this *I have had one goal—to give you back your life as the ongoing communion of ecstasy that it is.*

I have chosen to peel away the layers of dis-ease and untruth for the emergence of humanity by giving you back the absolute conviction that what I want for you is Love. I have made your road Home easy, My beloved ones. As easy as I possibly could. I know that within each and every one of you there is a memory, a memory of your SoulMate. There is a memory of a Love so personal and perfect that all you desire is manifested before you instantly. Oh, I have given you the assurance that all your secret dreams are real! There is a person who will love you in every way that you want to be loved. That person will shine upon you a sunshine of Love so warm and beautiful that you cannot help but blossom into the perfect expression of your true nature. All of this I promise you. *I ask of you only one thing. I ask that you will this to be so, and that you place Me in the center, the pinnacle of the triangle of perfect relationship.*

Yet even this, even this glorious Love, even this being who ever shows you the best of yourself, is only the beginning, for it is My hope that through the reclaiming of your Love you will also reclaim your life. Do you remember how often Jesus said, "I come to give you life, and that more abundantly?" (Trust Me, he said it continually.) He said this because humanity was then and is yet living only a tiny trickle of the great, magnificent LIFE that I have planned for you.

Now it is your turn. It is yours to pick up the Mantle of Christ to become the Christed Sons and Daughters of God. It is your time to reclaim your full truth. The doorway is your SoulMate, and this Love you share will ever be the center of your life, but it is only the beginning to living life abundantly.

Thus, with every touch, as you lay your hand upon your beloved's precious body, I ask you to affirm abundant life. Every moment that you look into his or her eyes, I ask you to stop and *feel* that moment. Let it penetrate your entire being. Let it fill your senses, wash you with light. And may you choose, beloved ones, to let each moment of Love be the doorway into your experience of the ecstasy of life. You are to become this ecstasy. You are meant to break through every barrier together, and thus to reclaim your passionate relationship with life.

I know that it is difficult to relate to streams of electrons and to the Moment of Creation. So I come to help you bring it all into the moments of your life. *I ask you to choose to awaken to life. To recognize that you are sleeping. To recognize that you are dreaming a shared dream of great limitation with the rest of humankind.* There are many reasons this dream has come to be a false reality for so many of My precious ones.

What matters now is that you wake. Reach your hand to your beloved SoulMate and choose to allow Love to bless and wake you. Here is the difference. In the dream, the pseudo reality you are living, you are never present. You are always adding new strands to the dream, calling it the future, calling it your needs, and most often calling it your fears. To wake from the dream, to experience life, you can only do so through the precious gift of being present in your moments, for I tell you that everything opens to Love. Everything. Your blessed hearts, your beloved bodies – every cell, every atom. Even Time will bow its head to Love. Even Time will release its hold as you cherish the moments of Love with your SoulMate. The moment you become present in the Eternal Moment in a vibration of Love, you will have access to your life. Your full life, your real life, your life more abundantly. As you are present in the moment, I ask you to look deeply into your beloved's eyes and experience the ecstasy. Allow yourselves to be totally consumed by joy. Stay here, carefully allowing only the experience of the Now Moment.

It may take practice. You may have to keep Making Love again and again! (Said with joy and a wash of Love – a cosmic smile.) But as you succeed you will become a unified experience of life, sinking together into the joyous union with All That Is. In other words, all of the chakras that I mentioned to you – the ones that extend below you and the ones above - will be awake to the joyous experience of that part of your life.

Please feel beyond the words, for I will show you. *I will show you that life is a passionate complete ecstatic connection with everything for you and your SoulMate. Once you are connected, if you then stay in the moment, then everything in Creation will be passionately in Love with you. Everything in Creation already is passionately in Love with you. You just don't notice. So the doorway of LoveMaking with your SoulMate will teach you how to notice life. That is being awakened from the dream.*

All of Creation is in glorious ecstatic Love with everything else. This, I ask you to know, to cherish, and to make it your goal to join the experience. It is not that everything is Love in some esoteric way. ***Dear ones,*** ***everything is in Love.*** To continually experience this passionate ecstatic union with everything is who you really are. Oh, that is "life more abundantly." That is what I mean by the ongoing Now Moment of Creation. Every single life form that is not cut off as you are, every single one, is continually experiencing this ecstatic union. It is the union with your SoulMate that will take you there. As you make Love, as you wake your cells, you come to understand that the tiny moment of orgasm you have experienced in sexual union is a millionth of a real orgasm between the two of you. Instead of a few cells in a few parts of your body currently deemed sexual, every single cell will be sharing in the orgasm experience. That in itself is a wonderful awakening. ***Suddenly you realize that you are ecstasy, not just having a*** ***moment of it.***

So first you will wake each other's bodies. You will pour your Love through your touch with two continual prayers: a prayer to Love your SoulMate more and more and more every moment. More purely. More passionately. More perfectly. With more joy, more tenderness, more and more ability to allow My Love to pour through you, lifting you as you then become My Love fully, in form. Then, secondly, the prayer of gratitude. Oh, with waves of joyous praise you must Love your beloved SoulMate. Praise every particle of his or her being, and see the amazing beauty, the magnificent qualities, the glorious reasons why every moment you Love him or her ever more. (If for some reason you are in your ego when you are together, then you must exert your will and pour forth such gratitude that ego is transcended.)

Oh, in these two prayers lies your transformation. For what you are meant to do together is to spiral upward into pure Love and ecstasy. As each of you look into the other's eyes, you will see the truth of your being, for your partner will be looking at you with such tender Love, also in the ecstasy of gratitude for your very presence. For perhaps the first time in your life, you will see yourself as I see you. In that moment you will have the truth shown to you in another's eyes, which is the Plan of Creation. You will be lifted out of the illusion. The hold of the lies, all of them, will be broken.

You will then do this for your partner, lifting him or her up and up, back and forth until you are perfect Love together in such high vibration that, reaching that frequency of Christ Light, every cell in your body opens like a butterfly to become impregnated by perfect light. Such opening also frees you from Time and from the dream. Your electrons switch, or weave together, and you are forever united on this plane. This is very important, for although you are experiencing a much higher than normal vibration, you are both still embodied (or at least one of you is), so you are thus bringing the Christ Light to Earth as Jesus did. It is not the same as someone reaching up until they essentially leave this plane. Instead, you are making Love physical, bringing Christ Light into all dimensions, and thus, making this path, this light, available here on Earth.

There is more! Isn't this wonderful?! That the very most glorious-beyond-imagining experience of Love is still not enough? Still not all of My gifts to you? Not yet the full truth of where you are going now?

Once your cells are open and you become the physical expression of Divine Masculine and Divine Feminine, then you are ready to expand your experience into Mine, into the truth of life. Once you are joined as the expression of pure Love and free of the illusion, you are fully in the Now Moment. All of your glorious chakras are now essentially your true sense organs of your real being, so that anything you turn your attention to, you experience. You experience a union of consciousness, meaning that you become one for that moment with whatever it is you thought of. One with the highest truth of their being. Thus if you were to think of an archangel you would become blended with that archangel. Completely. You would have the full, glorious, magnificent experience of being an archangel, and this experience would flow over you in waves of cosmic ecstasy. You can't yet even imagine what it would be like to BE an archangel, to literally hold forth the passionate Love of God, and literally be a flame of passion burning through the cosmos.

Imagine with a wave of your hand parting the clouds that bind whole planets, or delivering the living spirit of faith to those who need it, matching the intensity of your delivery perfectly to what each being can handle. Imagine being Archangel Michael! You would be, for as you turned your attention to him you would be blended in the Eternal Now. Both you and your SoulMate will experience it together.

Oh, that I could really show you. Oh, My beloved ones, choose to open to this endless joy, this complete passionate communion of Love that is your glorious natural state. Allow Me to give you a taste as you touch your SoulMate's body, be it physical or in the etheric body yet. Let this passionate Love of the moment throw open the doors of your being.

To continue in this awareness of your potential, what I described with the angels will be easy once all of your united being is open. What I have termed your higher chakras are your portals to experience on every level of the universe. The more you open to life and the more you move beyond Time, the more easily you will be wrapped in ecstatic communion with All That I Am (for of course that is all you are, too!).

If in your grand opening (a good play on words) you look together through your lower chakras that extend down below your feet, you would instantly have the glorious experience within yourself of every beauty-filled part of Nature. You would BE the growing tree with fingers in the gentle wind, and more than this, you would completely experience the ecstasy of the tree as it throws itself completely forth into sexual union with all it touches.

I tell you again that everything is ever part of Me as I experience the explosion of life. So the touch of the wind on the leaves of the tree will send waves of delicious, trembling, orgasmic ecstasy racing through its being.

Oh, beloved ones, humanity is one of only a few life forms that have chosen to turn away from this continual experience of bursting, tender, sweet, passionate pulsing union of life. I ask you to want it back! Want it back enough to break out of the hypnosis of your daily life. Begin here, in the sanctuary of your SoulMate Love to stop Time and to "be here now." Yes, you have all heard it, but no one is really doing it. Put forth the effort. Notice your life, and then promise.

Promise yourself and Me that you now deem sacred and most holy your LoveMaking — enough that you will experience every moment. Give your all – all your Love, appreciation, gratitude, tenderness. All your attention focused right there in every moment. This is why you must give up physical orgasm as the only goal of your sexuality. It keeps you bound in Time. It keeps you ever going toward something and thus you are not fully present in your moments.

The new movement of Love within you and the light it generates will draw more light into you. This will nourish and invigorate your cells way beyond what you accomplish through sleep. (Did you know this is why you have to sleep at night? To get out of the trap of Time enough that more light can get into your body – not to mention your mind!) So, as you begin to acknowledge your body and actually give it Love, you will need less sleep. I say this so you will be willing to experiment. If the only time you now have together is at night, be willing to use it freely without worrying you will be sleep deprived.

As you awaken into Love, awaken your entire being, including your bodies, your lives will change in many ways. As you come into the experience of the true ecstasy of life and you have moved beyond the dream, you will be surrounded by universal molten flowing Love. You will be able to reach out your hand (actually, more like reach out your mind) and simply claim for yourselves all good things.

Oh, please keep holding before your consciousness two things: the truth of your SoulMate and the truth of life, that everything is joined together in the experience of ecstasy. *Even you* – but you have to remember. You have to clear away the barrier, the membrane of Time, and of course any false feelings (anything below Love), and you will be there. Imagine, dear ones, joined together with your SoulMate in the constant assurance of My Love (so constant I will manifest it in front of you the moment you allow Me to), experiencing the glorious, pulsing, ecstatic union with everything you encounter.

This awakening may be fast or slow, but it will be, for it is our Will. Whether or not you remember it, we planned this reunion. We agreed that once you were individualized you would return. The Tree of Life would be whole again. That Tree is you, with all your chakras awakened – those joining you with Nature and those joining you with all higher realms. It is the full experience of you as the "center of the Garden." You are the center. The center of Creation. The Heart of All I Am. You are beautiful beyond compare.

Oh, My sweet ones, you are waking up at last. So long you have lain in your beds and dreamed, the angels gathered at your bedside. I have held you tenderly in the safety of My consciousness. Beside you have been your precious friends, the allies of your dream world, beings of Nature, animals and elves, dwarfs and fairies, giving you reminders, though some of you have laughed at "fairy tales."

I am so ready to see your faces when you awake. Oh, ready to watch your eyes light up, your hearts swell in gratitude and your every cell be melted in the tenderness of Love. I am ready. So I come to prepare you for waking. To remind you that you have always slept in the arms of your beloved SoulMate. For though you imagined I could leave you, that I could deem you lonely, bereft, living in pain - it is not true. What loving parent would ever want that for her/his children? NONE. And I Am the Great Parent whose very heart bears you, wrapped within My tender Love.

"It's time to wake up," I am whispering. Your cells are hearing Me. Your atoms are dancing in excitement. All that remains is for you to arise, to wipe the sleep from your eyes and to remember. Truly, just as you dream the most amazing things in your current human sleep, when you wake you shake your head at the things your mind creates. It is the same, beloved ones. It is the same. When you wake you will have no trouble seeing that you have been dreaming.

As you know, you accomplish this now when you die to this Earth life and awake on the other side. But here is the difference. These cells you wear are still your Love. They are frozen, true, but you cannot leave them behind. If you think about it you will understand that you must honor and retain and return to Love with every part of you intact. You cannot leave the physical plane, for you are its life. You are animating it, and you must lift it back into the awakened communion with your awakened heart. And that is what we are doing. You will come to see the power of these words and you will come to feel this truth even more powerfully yet.

You are coming back to consciousness, remembering your SoulMate. So wherever the experience of that part of your consciousness has been, it is now on its path of awakening to you, remembering you as you remember, too. Then together you must awaken every part of yourselves, rejoin in Love and thus reclaim the entire experience.

So we say you will "take these bodies with you," but in truth of course, they always have been with you. You have simply been asleep and since the only time you remembered was between lives (between dreams!), you thought your bodies were not part of it.

Now I must say one last and crucial thing. I have been focusing here on your awakening, for I know that the moment you even glimpse outside the dream, you will know the truth of life, that it truly is only by giving that you receive. You will learn this with your SoulMate. You will learn it and learn it and learn it – for if you forget you will "lose altitude" immediately. So, quickly or slowly, you will incorporate giving on all levels in every direction and dimension, in order to receive. First you will start by giving to each other, both Love and gratitude. Then quickly you will come to understand that you are connected to everything. Every time you make it into the true experience of the moment, you will flash through into a communion of Love in which you are completely one with All That Is.

If your heart is open, giving will take care of itself, for an open heart is a giving heart. And thus I give you a measure of your freedom. Is it your greatest joy to give? If the answer is "yes," then to that degree you are in your heart. In Love.

Moving beyond the dream. If the answer (honestly) is "no," to that degree you are still in your ego. It is that simple.

As it becomes your greatest joy to give, then the door is open for Love in its passionate, beautiful molten state to pour through you. To that same degree, you are then available for all those beings so tenderly serving the awakening of humanity. If you begin the flow by the use of your Will (deciding to give), they can all rush forth to use you, for your giving creates a flow that opens a vortex outside of the dream. Into this opening the angels and masters and all those who are helping can pour in "missing ingredients" to bring health and life to the whole of humanity.

I give you no more instruction for LoveMaking than these here given, because you must use your creativity. How you touch your SoulMate, how you pour your Love, your delight, your energy to wake the beloved cells and atoms of their body – it's up to you.

How you use your generated energy – to lift yourselves, to bless the world, to rejoin the orgasmic moment of Creation – this will be your experiment for you are co-creators, and you are in Love. Thus you must communicate this Love with each other. You can ask your beloved for what you need, for you have an intuitive connection, of course, to the cells of your body, and they will tell you what they want and where they are in the waking process.

The more you practice Love in the moment, the more clearly each of you will know. You will know what your partner needs. You will know what you need. You will know how much I Love you, that you are everything to Me. You are My progeny, as well as being My own heart, so if nothing else you can always explore how a perfectly loving parent would love you and would treat every part of your experience.

I will continue, of course, giving you keys to this awakening. Keys to communication both within (with the cells) and without (with the cosmos). I will continue to raise your consciousness of Sacred Sexuality. So the ending of this manuscript is certainly not an end to anything other than a chosen size for a book!

I love you. Passionately. When you understand the passion of God, you will understand yourselves. I can promise you that even those who seem so soft and gentle and full of sweet light (like Mary) ARE living in a passionate exaltation of life. Yet it is expressed perfectly through their being. Of course, as you know, each and every one of My Creations is unique. Each and every one of you has a place in Creation, a role to fill, an expansion of Love that no one else can accomplish. So My precious ones, please cherish your expression of Love and vow to bring it forth now.

TO THE READER

If you resonate strongly with what you have just read, please know that there are more books of Messages from God that continue the thrilling journey to the Twin Flame and Christ consciousness. *Say YES to Love, God's Guidance to LightWorkers* and *Say YES to Love, God Leads Humanity Toward Christ Conscious* are available for purchase on our website, www.circleoflight.net, and *Say YES to Love, Giving Birth to the Christ Light* is in the process of publication.

The pages that follow contain two powerful communications, personal to each of us, given through the Messages from God. **Dissolving Impediments to Opening the Heart** came as a meditation, given to assist us in releasing any blocks to an open heart and to accelerate reunion with our SoulMate. This is also available as a CD, in an expanded form, and can be ordered at our website (#6 in the CD list). **A Letter from God to Humanity on Creating a World of Love** is included here in response to God's request for the widest possible distribution of this Message. It can also be obtained on CD, by writing to our email, connect@circleoflight.net.

We invite you to join our Spiritual Family. Our active Circle of Light website, www.circleoflight.net, contains much information including excerpts and complete Messages from God on many subjects. You may sign up for our email list for bi-monthly Messages from God and Newsletters, and you may also place yourself on the list for transcripts of our Tuesday evening meditation Circle (Tuesday Circle). CDs of all our meditations are also available on the website (see Tuesday Circle Meditations).

Circle of Light Workshops are a calling to Twin Flame hearts in service --LightWorkers who feel resonance with these Messages and have come into the world to lift it back to Love. Descriptions and pictures of our workshops are also on our website. With open hearts we call you to explore all of this.

May you live with an open heart in a world of Love every moment.

The Team at Circle of Light

Dissolving Impediments
To Opening The Heart

The following Meditation on *Dissolving Impediments to Opening the Heart* was given through Yael Powell at Circle of Light on Tuesday November 19, 2002, during a group meeting. An expanded version given on April 24, 2004 is available as a CD on our website, for those who prefer to listen.

Once you have done this Meditation and established this connection with God, heart's beliefs will arise and be shown to you. If you will give them to God, God will remove them.

You may re-experience briefly in your mind and emotions the situations that created these impediments, even with some discomfort. This is the "replay" as the removal is occurring. If this occurs, know that it is of the past, and do not be concerned. Simply pray gratitude, giving thanks for the fact that all blockages to your completely open heart are now being removed. Reading the excerpt from the Messages from God at the end of the Meditation will clarify this.

As you do the Meditation, read a paragraph, and then close your eyes and allow time to completely absorb the experience.

Meditation On Dissolving Impediments To Opening The Heart

Begin by taking deep breaths, sinking into your heart with all of your consciousness. With every breath in, open your heart, larger and larger and larger. As you breathe in and your heart opens, feel yourself connecting to the All of God, the great ocean of Love, vibrant and alive, vast, yet tender.

So now you have a gloriously open heart connected to the All of Love. The vast, the un-manifest. And now you feel that ocean of God's Love permeating your being and funneling through your heart. Not just your physical heart, of course, but the heart of Love that you are. With every out-breath, God pours through you to touch and love manifested life.

We are aware of ourselves now as that point where God loves through us. Be conscious of how it feels as Love pours through you. Feel how it blesses, how it kisses every cell of your body, how it illuminates every particle of Love that you are, how it resonates with the light that is in every atom, with the life that you are. How does it feel to be the very heart of God?

Breathe in, becoming the open heart, communing with the All of Love. Breathe out as Love pours through the opening that is you and God's Love comes into the world. Notice how it feels to be touched by this Love, to be its vehicle, its vessel. Allow the Love to pour through you and your mind to notice, AFTER the fact. Notice, if you can, how this Love honors the truth of who you are, your existence.

As you feel this Love pouring through you, keep expanding in your awareness of the heart that you are. Expanding until there is nothing else. No personality, no body, only the glorious opening for Love. Feel the celebration of life, exaltation, joy as that Love pours through you. Notice that there is only Love, washing through you, pouring through you, rushing through you, without discrimination. It doesn't go some places and not to others. It doesn't find some lives worthy and others not. It just pours through you. All of life manifest is being loved through us. The rushing, dancing river of living Love, pouring through the heart of God we are.

Now placing our consciousness right at that point that is the opening of our heart, the place where God's Love pours through, the window pane of our spirit – the heart – allow to rise up before this opening something that restricts the passage of this Love — something that is a belief or a part of who you think you are, something that needs the forgiveness of letting go. Allow it to rise up from within from the wisdom that God is with you. Hold it there in front of the opening that is your heart.

Now, breathing in – connect to the glorious All of the Love of God and allow that Love pouring through your heart to love that flaw, that part that needs releasing. To love it, to love it, to pour that Love upon it with passion and with tenderness, all the urgency of the river of life, reaching through to lift it up, to dissolve its hold on your heart. Love washes it tenderly until you see it dissolving, until where there was a blockage, there is only living Love. Know that anything exposed to this Love can only dissolve, its energy freed at last.

And now, breathing in, you are held within the All of God. You are held in Love so magnificent that you are filled with joy and love so tender that you are sure in every fiber of your being of God's personal support of you. You are suspended in abundance and perfection – the perfection of God's Love for you. You are resting in the ocean of God and you are filled with a clarity you have never known – the you are filled with a clarity you have never known – the experience of how precisely God shows you your unique beauty, the truth of your creation. This glorious all-encompassing, personal yet limitless Love of God reveals to you the full capacity of your heart, so that now…

Breathing out, God's Love now flows through you completely unimpeded. The opening that is the center of your being, the great heart that you are is filled with ecstasy because now you are aware that this very same tender uplifting, deeply personal Love of God you have experienced, can pour through your heart. In this way God may reach others through the sacred opening for Love that you are. The "window-pane" of your spirit, the center of your being, your heart, is crystal clear.

Breathing in, you feel the sweet support of the All of God, reflecting to you your truest self. Breathing out, you know yourself as the clear unimpeded heart through which God now perfectly loves the world. Every person, every plant, every particle of energy – God will love them through you. And as divine Love is ever moving through you, you will be giving beyond any thought or desire to receive. Just so will you truly receive all that you give, which is now all that God gives through you, multiplied and delivered to your open and accepting heart.

Now you have the assurance that all impediments will be removed from your heart by God. So you can simply rest in this assurance – that God will do the work of Love in and through you now in each and every moment.

Commentary on Dissolving Impediments
To Opening The Heart

Excerpt from *The Messages from God*
Through Yaël Powell, Circle of Light
November 24, 2002

"The impediments before your heart, any one of you, unravel like a skein of wool when the Love hits it, and unraveling, they do 'replay' themselves. They engage the projector, pull down the screen and play a movie in your mind. For, of course, this is what life in the ego really is – billions of unraveling 'movies' playing out the mind's beliefs, over and over, as the light of My Love seeks entry.

"Yet you can know, you who now begin to come to the central point consciously, that the more you stay out of your mind, the fewer new movies' you create, and soon (sooner than you think), there won't be any 'movie reels' left to play.

"When you say, 'Yes,' to Love, you are saying that you are willing to dissolve those impediments. To let the light of My Love into the movie theatre. Thus, for you who see your lives becoming beauty, the reflection of your heart — you can know that if suddenly you are 'in the play' again, it IS the clearing out of those things cluttering up the heart space, those things that 'push the pendulum' so that it swings away from the center point. Especially if you are choosing to accept the tools given [the above Meditation], then you can positively know this is the case, and that it won't take long and you will be able to remain in the stillness of My Love, allowing Me to live every moment through you."

A Letter From God to Humanity On Creating A World Of Love

Through Yael and Doug Powell
February 25, 2003

My beloved ones, humanity, I pour this to you with My tender Love, upon streams of light, to touch your waiting hearts. With it come the keys to your remembrance. The remembrance of your beauty and of all the ways I made you in My image. And remembrance of the truth of Love, how every human heart was born in Love and every human being is a child of God. And the remembrance that your heart is our connection and that through it lives your co-creative power. Through it comes your treasure; all the gifts I give to you forever. Through it you will now remember and find yourselves awaking to the truth of Love you are.

How I love you! You are truly the greatest of all miracles. You are My own heart, alive and in embodiment, ready to expand, to ever go forth to give the Love you are. You make Love vibrant, surprising, new. Only you, beloved ones, My precious glorious children, only you can go forth in breathless anticipation and see the Love I Am with a new perspective. Have you not marveled at your wonderful curiosity? At how insatiably you go forward to meet and greet the world? And how deeply you are moved by every expansion of beauty? This is the miracle of your co-creative heart.

My Will for you, all of you, every sweet magnificent golden child of God, is a world of peace and a life of plenty. By looking at Me, you can have these things.

Your heart is the source of your power, your treasure, your identity, your life. Your heart is connected to Me forever. And through your heart you will receive your blessings, the treasures of joy and Love and ever greater abundance that I have waiting for you. Oh! It is My heart's true desire to deliver to you the very keys to heaven that you may live heaven here on Earth, yes, and everywhere you are for all eternity. All that is necessary is for you to return to your heart to find the joy in life that contains the heart's true resonance and the cornucopia of every good, which shall pour forth before you as your life and your world.

I Am a God of Love, dear ones. Forever and forever. There is nothing but Love in Me. Let your heart stir in its remembrance of the great truth, for on it rests the salvation of this precious world and your thousand years of peace that, truly, goes on forever. You have known this, somewhere deep inside. You have known that I Am Love and that all of this before you did not make sense. All the wars and illnesses, the brothers turning upon their brothers, the poverty, the pain, even ageing and death. Oh, dear ones, I have heard you as you cried out in the dark night of your soul for answers. How every single one of you has asked the question, "If God loves us, why would God create children who have cancer and whole peoples who are starving; so emaciated they already look like skeletons?" It did not seem right to you. This, dear ones, was the message of your heart seeking to show you the truth. And when you have asked, "God, what is my purpose, the meaning of my life?" you have been responding to the nudging of your heart. But some, not hearing their hearts, have turned away, believing I could not be a loving parent to My children if I created such a world of horrors.

Now it is time for the truth. You are ready. And for those of you who read this and already know this, I ask you to deepen your commitment to the living of it, and to pass this on to My other precious children. For those of you who read this and find it inconceivable, I ask you to drop into a focus on your heart for a moment and just allow this to be a possibility. Then pass it on to others – that each hand, each set of eyes, each heart that comes in contact with this letter written in light may also take a moment to allow this possibility to be planted in their life.

Beloved ones, I love you. I love you with a Love as great as the very cosmos. I love you with a joy in your existence that pours forth greater in every moment. I love you as the very heart within Me. I love you, and My Love never wavers, never changes, never ever stops. I long for you to know this, to feel our sweet communion. I long to lay before you all the treasures of creation. You are Mine. Now. And Now. Forever. And nothing can ever change this. It is a fact of your existence.

I did not create this world of pain. You did. You did this when you chose to believe in good, in Love, **and** in something else, which you named the opposite of Love.
Call it the moment in the Garden when you ate the fruit of good and evil. Call it the first judgment. Whatever you call it, beloved ones, it is your own creation. And you set yourselves up as being able to decide which was which and thus began this world of duality, of light *and* dark, of Love and anti-Love. But, precious humanity, I Am only Love. And living in Me, you, too, are only Love. So you had to create a false world, a pretend place where darkness could exist, because it cannot exist in that which is ever and only light, which I Am.

You have wandered in the desert of your co-creative minds ever since. For if your heart, connected to Me, knows the truth of only Love, then you had to find another way to view a dual scenario – and thus evolved the tool of your minds.

Call it the moment in the Garden when you ate the fruit of good and evil. Call it the first judgment. Whatever you call it, beloved ones, it is your own creation. And you set yourselves up as being able to decide which was which and thus began this world of duality, of light *and* dark, of Love and anti-Love. But, precious humanity, I Am only Love. And living in Me, you, too, are only Love. So you had to create a false world, a pretend place where darkness could exist, because it cannot exist in that which is ever and only light, which I Am.

You have wandered in the desert of your co-creative minds ever since. For if your heart, connected to Me, knows the truth of only Love, then you had to find another way to view a dual scenario – and thus evolved the tool of your minds.

Oh, dear ones, I do not intend to go into lengthy explanations. All I come to say to you is that you are only Love. And that the more you choose to live through your heart, the more and more clearly you'll see the world as it really is. The more you will experience that true Love of God, the Love that I hold you in each and every moment.

Today you live in a world on the brink of war, a world filled with negativity and so much pain that you have to numb yourselves to survive. So you have nothing to lose by putting to the test what I now show you.

If you know that I Am only Love, then you must know that I Am ever holding for you the world of your inheritance, the world of joyous ecstasy and glorious abundance. You know that I Am not a power you can call on for overcoming darkness, for darkness is not in Me. You know that any moment you connect with Me you connect with the Love and perfection I have always held for you and always will. I Am unchanging Love. In the truth of this Love there is no negativity.

Then what about this world of pain before you? What of the wars and rumors of wars? What of the fear and all the experiences that keep happening in your life? They are you, dreaming, beloved one. They are you lost within the million threads of possibility streaming from your decision to believe in good *and* evil. And just as you dream in the night and your dreams feel real, so it is with this world. So very real and filled with pain, it feels.

There is another way to live. It is to stand before this world of lies each morning and to choose to live in only Love. To consciously reject the illusion of the judgment that there is good and evil. To place your Will in Mine and ask that I lift you up enough that you can see the difference. The difference between the truth of Love that lives within your heart and this world of swirling negativity that is alive within your mind.

And once you know that I Am Love and you are ever alive in Me, then you shall truly walk through this world in peace. When you know your home is Me and you affirm the heart, you could walk through a war-torn countryside with bombs falling all around you and know that none could touch you, and none would touch our home.

I will answer your questions. "What about the others?" your heart cries out. "What good is it if I am safe in you, God, if all around me people are in misery?" Beloved ones, the answer is this: as you clear the dream, as you return your Will to Me, as you walk within the truth of the Love we are together, then around you there becomes an aura of peace; a great ball of light comes forth as the living truth of Love you are becoming. At first it may only clear *your* life of the illusion, as your faith in Love restores you to the heaven you belong in, and as, choice-by-choice and day-by-day, you turn to Me for your identity and not to the world you have believed is outside of choice-by-choice and day-by-day, you turn to Me for your identity and not to the world you have believed is outside of you. But every day that light grows – exactly as would happen if you turn on a physical light in a dark closet full of scary shapes. The light fills every space – there is no darkness left – and everything that seemed to be so menacing becomes something neutral. Something you can change by moving out the old furniture, or something that you at least know is harmless.

Thus, as you grow in your ability to stay attuned to Me, to choose the world that is your birthright as a child of God, the greater the circumference of the light that surrounds you. First it begins to light up your neighbors. Suddenly they can see that there are no terrifying things lurking in their lives; that they are free to choose to be happy, to have joy. And with every moment that you spend in communion with the truth of your heart, the greater is that light of truth around you...until you affect the neighborhood and then the town you live in, and the county, then the state in which you live. Until ultimately you will do as Jesus did: everywhere you are, people will see their truth as Love, and knowing this with all their heart they will leave their illnesses, their problems and their strife behind – simply from experiencing the power of your light as you live your life as only Love.

Then as others do the same, soon you'll walk into the world and the illusion of negativity will have to fall away. You will have "turned on the light in the theater," that which you call the world, and all who had believed life was a battle will suddenly be freed.

In your Western world, there is a passage in the Bible from he who came to show you the way to the heart's truth: "You cannot serve both God and mammon." This is exactly what it means. You cannot believe in a world of good and evil and also seek to create a life of Love. For from within the dream of duality every choice for Love contains its opposite.

Beloved ones, if this speaks to you, if something stirs within your heart (or, of course, if you cry out, "Oh, I know this!"), then you are here to show the way. Here to see My face, My Love, in every human being, no matter the part they now play within the dream of good and evil, of Love and anti-Love. You are here to build the New, to bring forth the heaven of living Love in which you are ever meant to live. Turn to Me and daily, moment by precious moment, I will show you who you are: a child of Love so beautiful that your cloak is made of stars, your heart is a living sun lighting up the darkness and revealing only light.

Give Me your Will, let Me lift you so you can see each moment the unity of Love. How all creation is My being and every part, magnificent and joyous, dances in a swirl of sweet exploding life. I will help you see beyond duality, beyond the veil within which lives the dream of separation being dreamed by My children. I Am only Love. And your heart is the key to the treasures held for you beyond time. Time – the illusory creation coming forth from "fitting into experience" a pendulum of good and bad experience.

Beloved ones, I speak to you whose hearts have known, have known deep inside that I would not create such a world as this you see before you. It can be easy to disengage, but you've lived the illusion for a long time. Thus can you assist each other in this. Assist each other in placing your attention on your hearts and using the power of Love you find there to infuse the world you want, not the world that's passing, the world of so much pain. You are co-creators. Made in My image, remember? It is true. You are made in My image and thus do you manifest the beliefs of your heart. Remember, the heart is where we are connected, so all the power, all the light, all the Love I pour to you comes directly and unfailingly to and through your heart. I Am Creator; I Am Love expanding through you.

And My covenant with you, My children, is that I shall always and forever grant your heart's desires. This is the promise given to each of you at the moment of your creation as children of the Love I Am. So if deep in your heart you are afraid, if you believe your heart is broken (pay attention to these words), if you are afraid that Love will hurt you, if you keep yourself protected, if you are waiting every moment for "the other shoe to drop," if you feel the world is hopeless, if you feel that life's not worth it, if you feel the world's about to end, be it from polluting it to death or from chaos and war, these deep "ways you feel" about your life – these are your heart's beliefs. And thus, beloved ones, *by our covenant* they shall manifest before you. For as the Love I Am comes pouring to you, whatever is held before the opening of your heart is what Love shall bring to life, shall help you co-create.

Thus you see that, if you stand before the White House with anger in your heart, with belief that nothing changes, that government is corrupt, and, worst of all, if you hold hatred there, within the temple of God that you are, then that, dear ones, is what you shall have more of.

You are the prize of the universe – the heart of God gone forth to create. There is really only Love to create with. But if you choose Love and anti-Love, you turn your face away from Love and, peering into the world you've made, you look for your identity. Oh, precious ones, don't find it there! Please wake into the truth of Love. Place your every resource with your true and glorious heart. I promise you that Love is the only power. And that, truly, it is the heart with which you shall always create what you experience, be it now, on Earth, or later, "after death." There is no progression, no good and bad, no better and best. There is only the truth of Love or the dream of separation.

If you can make this leap, you are those who bridge heaven and Earth, who begin to reclaim the paradise you never really left. But if you cannot, then please do continue on growing in your faith in Love. It is good to pray for peace, for even though it contains the belief in its opposite, for the moments you are focusing on Love you are using your co-creative consciousness to lift you ever closer to the unity of Love. It is best, however (and I use these terms because they are relevant here), it is the true way, the way that Jesus came to show you, to see only Love. To place every bit of the power of your heart upon the paradise of Love that this Earth is in truth, giving none of your energy to the illusion that I can ever create anything but Love.

Do you see? Do you see how this must be a fantasy if in Me darkness does not exist? If I Am All That Is, which I Am, then nowhere in Creation is there anything but Love. Oh, dear ones, this I promise you. You were created in Love; made as a glorious reproduction of what I Am as Creator. You thus came forth, truly, as Twin Flames, the forces of the Divine. Ocean of Love, Divine Feminine, and the great movement of My Will upon it, Divine Masculine. Born as one with two points of conscious Love, you forever exist in a grand unity of Love, sparking together to co-create more Love.

I call you home. Home to the unity of Love I Am and that you are in Me. Every thought for peace, every prayer has value, and every act of service in Love's name to another is a star in the night of this "pocket of duality." But the real service for which many of you have come is to join together, heart after heart, in the conviction of the truth of only Love and, forming a net of your great auras of light, to lift the world free of the reversal caused by humanity's belief in good and evil.

Thank you, beloved one, for reading this. Do you feel My living presence in your heart? Do you see the light behind these words, the packages of Love I now deliver? Then you are called, beloved one. Called to remember a world of only Love. Called to place this vision before you until it sinks into your heart and becomes your one desire: to return to My children their birthright. You have angels all around you. Your hands are being held, finger of light to finger of light, by the masters who go before you to pave the way. Your every affirmation of the world of Love you choose is heralded by archangels as they trumpet across the heavens, "A child of God awakes! A child of God awakes!" And choruses of beings, living stars greater than your sun, carry forth the message that the whole of Love I Am is filled with rejoicing. For every child of God who returns heals those many lives of the dreams of anti-Love that sprang forth from their creative heart. And the whole of the cosmos is glad, because a hole in My heart, caused by your facing away into "darkness," is healed. The heart of God is mended, ah, but more than this: the Love I Am goes forth again as you to create new things for us to love together.

I Am calling. You can hear Me. It won't be long now, beloved ones.

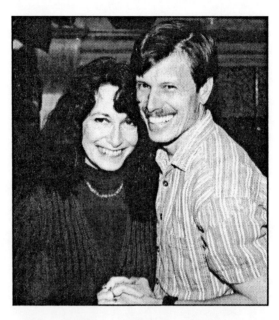

ABOUT YAEL AND DOUG POWELL
AND CIRCLE OF LIGHT

Yael and Doug Powell live at Circle of Light, their spiritual center in Eureka Springs, Arkansas, that looks out over Beaver Lake and the Ozark Mountains. Both Yael and Doug are ordained ministers, and the lovely Chapel at Circle of Light is the frequent scene of beautiful sacred weddings.

Yael spends a good deal of her time in bed as a result of pain from a severe physical disability. Her "up-time" is spent officiating at weddings or receiving the Messages from God in meditation. Doug is an artist and skilled craftsman at pottery and woodworking. If it is windy, you'll definitely find him at his lifelong passion – sailing! Shanna Mac Lean, compiler and editor of the Messages, also lives at Circle of Light. If not at the computer, she can be found in the organic vegetable garden.

Completing the Circle of Light family are their wonderful animal companions. Christos (boy) and Angel (girl) are their two beloved Pomeranians. Ariel (Duff Duff) is a pure white cat who has been with Yael and Doug for 17 years. He mostly frequents the garden and occasionally attends a wedding. Then there is Magic Cat, of course with his entourage -- his SoulMate, Magic's Love (Love, for short); and their sister Sweetheart, Shanna's "Sweetie." These babies celebrated their first birthday on July 24, 2004, and it would be no exaggeration to say that they rule the household.

CIRCLE OF LIGHT ORDER FORM
Say "Yes" to Love Series

Please send the following:

_____ copies of God Explains Soulmates @ $11 _____($3 S&H)

_____ copies of God Unveils SoulMate Love & Sacred Sexuality @ $20.00 _____ ($3.50 S&H)

_____ copies of God's Guidance to LightWorkers @ $ 14 _____($3 S&H)

_____ copies of God Leads Humanity Toward Christ Consciousness @ $16 _____($3 S&H)

_____ copies of Magic Cat Explains Creation! @ $16 _____($3 S&H)

_____ copies of Giving Birth to the Christ Light @ $16 _____($3 S&H)

Name: _____

Address: _____

City: _____State:_____ Zip Code:_____

To use credit cards, please go to our web site www.circleoflight.net OR you may fax your order with credit card to (479) 253-2880.

Name on card: _____

CC#: _____ Exp date:_____

If you would like to be on our email list and receive bi-monthly Messages from God, please fill out the following:

Email address: _____

Circle of Light
3969 Mundell Road, Eureka Springs, Arkansas 72631
www.circleoflight.net • www.unitingtwinflames.com
connect@circleoflight.net
1-866-629-9894 Toll Free or 479-253-6832, 2774